"If you want a reassuring guide, one th~
reminds you of your inner wisdom a
ing path, get this book and keep it as
feel like you are making a friend, beca
soul friendship—with each other, with   with the
planet.

This book is both radical and authentic. Radical because it
deeply connects us to our roots in community and the Earth.
Authentic in its personal stories, honesty, and constant gentle
reminders to be good to ourselves. *The Circle of Healing* builds
important bridges, a welcome gift helping us usher in the
healing century."

—K. Lauren de Boer, editor, *EarthLight Magazine*

"A wonderful portal to enter, or continue on, the road of personal growth and development. Each page brims with practical
nuggets of wisdom. Read a chapter a day and allow Holt's
concepts and practices based upon self-regulation to nurture
the wholeness within. Inspiring reading for anyone who wants
to enter and stay in the circle of healing."

—Erik Peper, Ph.D., Director, Institute for Holistic Healing
Studies, San Francisco State University; co-author, *Creating
Wholeness* and *Healthy Computing with Muscle Biofeedback*

"Gems of wisdom on every page . . . simply magnificent.
Philosophy, trauma recovery, nature, and much more. Holt
writes with humor, depth, and amazing perceptiveness. She
takes the wisdom of great philosophers, ancient and modern,
and adds to the triumph of the human spirit through her
own spiritual journey of healing. A book that could be life-
changing!"

—Shel Horowitz, author, environmental activist, and
founder of Save The Mountain

The Circle of Healing

for Christian
with all the blessings
of the Circle —

Cathy Holt

The *Circle of* *Healing*

Deepening Our Connections with Self, Others, and Nature

Cathy Holt

Talking Birds
Press

Published by:
TALKING BIRDS PRESS
P. O. Box 13073
Berkeley, CA 94712
1-800-404-9492

Printed on **Vanguard Recycled Plus,** ™ a virgin-fiber-free paper
consisting of 90 percent post-consumer waste and 10 percent hemp,
acid free and processed chlorine free, with soy-based ink

Printed in the United States of America

Cover mandala: "The Winged Ones" by Augusta Lucas-Andreae
Cover design by Pete Masterson
Text design by Diana Young

Publisher's Cataloging-in-Publication
(Provided by Quality Books, Inc.)

Holt, Catherine F.
    The circle of healing : deepening our connections
    with self, others, and nature / by Cathy Holt. -- 1st ed.
    p. cm.
    LCCN: 00-90173
    ISBN: 0-9677777-0-4

    1. Mental healing. 2. Self-actualization
(Psychology) 3. Holistic medicine. I. Title

RZ400.H65 2000   615.8'52
               QBI00-482

This book is dedicated to
my mother, Louisa Pinkham Holt Howe,
and to my father, Robert Holt,
with oceans of love and gratitude.

Acknowledgements

This book was birthed by many midwives, many people in my circle of support. My mother, Louisa Howe, provided many of the ideas in the chapter on judgments. My father, Robert Holt, believed in me, and edited my book—twice! My good friend Augusta Lucas-Andreae provided the beautiful mandala on the cover, entitled "The Winged Ones." Ria Pflaum-Murphy reminded me to think big, and took me for walks up into the hills when I needed to regain perspective! Dennis Rivers and Miki Kashtan introduced me to compassionate communication. My yoga teacher, Rodney Yee, taught me to let my heart lead instead of my head. My wonderfully resourceful editor, Diana Young, helped and encouraged me through the rough spots. My ex-husband, Dennis DiBartolomeo, patiently taught me the computer skills I needed to write this book. David Wheeler, age 5, offered love and inspiration. For all their solidarity, friendship, and humor, I appreciate my "Year to Live" group: Donna Landon, Marshall McComb, Freya Hermanson, Kate O'Malley, and Al Bettles. Thanks also to my community circle: Miki, Monica, Ken, Etta, Dick, Susan, Al, Diana, and Irene. Many, many other friends read drafts and offered insightful comments.

Others in my circle of support include all those teachers who have most influenced me: Angeles Arrien, Brooke Medicine Eagle, Thich Nhat Hanh, Joanna Macy, John Seed, Erik Peper, Stephen Levine, Michael Cohen, Sun Bear, Pat Norris, Martin Rossman, Barbara Sher, Lawrence LeShan, Tim Corcoran, Marshall Rosenberg, Joanne Lauck, Jerry Jampolsky, Aeeshah Ababio, Leslie Gray, Dick Roy, ChoQosh Au-Ho-Oh, Serge King.

My thanks to all these allies!

Contents

Everything the Power of the world does is done in a circle. The sky is round, and I have heard that the earth is round like a ball, and so are all the stars. The wind, in its greatest power, whirls. Birds build their nests in circles, for theirs is the same religion as ours. The sun comes forth and goes down again in a circle. The moon does the same, and both are round. Even the seasons form a great circle in their changing, and always come back again to where they were. The life of a man is a circle from childhood to childhood, and so it is in everything where power moves.

—Black Elk

Introduction

The circle of healing represents the truth that we are not healed alone, but through joining. The circle is the symbol of wholeness. It is a sacred womb in which visions can be nurtured. In Native American traditions, it represents the life cycle, as well as the sacred hoop of life. Nature moves in circles and seasonal cycles, not in lines and rows. Michael Bridge, a local poet, observes:

> We live in square houses lined up in rows and
> blocks laid out in cities and towns that are more
> like waffle grids than living things because we are
> crazy and we don't know what to do about it.

In the great cycles of nature, we experience that whatever we do to another is done to us. Pollution of rivers and oceans will soon foul the watery cells of our own bodies; restoration of a natural area helps restore us.

When we sit in a circle, everyone is equidistant from the middle; all have an equal voice. "If there is a performance in the center, or a jewel in the center, or a fire in the center, or a problem in the center, we are all equally near or equally far away," says Anthea Francine, a therapist and teacher. Since no one has more power, each person draws on his or her own authority. The circle is a container for everything. Being at the same time the symbol for nothing (zero) and for wholeness or completion, the circle symbolizes the unity of opposites. I invite you to join me in this circle.

According to Caroline Myss, author of *Anatomy of the Spirit*, "The perception that time and life are linear experiences handicaps the healing process." Let's trade in straight-ahead tunnel vision for a holistic, 360-degree vision. Originally I had thought of healing in a linear way, as a path or a journey. That implies having to leave where we are right now and seek wholeness elsewhere. I have come to see that a major part of my healing lies in accepting that who I am, where I am right now is good enough. So what if I have had an embarrassingly long apprenticeship!

This book was organically grown. No pesticides! It evolved gradually over time from my struggles toward healing. Painful experiences became rich compost from which paragraphs sprouted. At first I wrote short handouts to give to friends and biofeedback clients at the clinic where I was working. When I had a few of these, I assembled them into a little booklet with the help of the computer and the xerox machine. Whenever I added more sections or expanded on a theme, I printed up a new edition to give away. New sections would emerge out of my own life experience. Sometimes a whole new branch would be added, sometimes it seemed that the roots simply went deeper or the trunk grew a little thicker. Nature has gently insisted that I make this book ever mossier, greener, and filled with bird trills.

Many stories from my life are woven into this book. Personal stories have always engaged me more fully than abstract statements; perhaps they speak to both halves of my brain. Our life experiences are multileveled and rich in meanings. There are stories like "Alice in Wonderland," as well as many fairy tales and myths that appeal to both children and adults because they offer different, important life messages to each.

Recording these personal stories and insights has been part of my healing process by deepening my level of awareness. What I teach is what I most need to learn. The chapter on judgments is the longest because I've needed to work on healing from the sickness of judgmentalism.

One of my intentions in this book is honesty. My aim is to tell the truth about myself without blame or self-judgment, a very healing practice I learned from Angeles Arrien. In revealing more of myself, I'm choosing not to try to look better than I really am. I'm a long way from following all of the wonderful practices that I know are helpful for me. And my healing process is still ongoing. Sometimes I spend several months at a time barking up the wrong tree. It was a great relief to realize that, even though I often overeat and underbreathe, I still have something to offer. Part of my personal song to sing is the sigh of relief!

How might you use this book? I suggest that you read a little bit at a time, in whatever order appeals to you. The sequence of the chapters is intuitive rather than linear. Read when you feel stuck, angry, hopeless. Read a few pages right before bed, and/or first thing in the morning. Open it at random and read what is there.

This book offers hope, self-help strategies, and some different perspectives to people who are struggling with the limitations of the current medical establishment in dealing with their crises. Most of all, this is a book about nature: coming home to our true nature, and letting nature guide and heal us. I hope that some of these ideas and methods that have helped me may be of use to you.

Beginning to Heal

Health is inner peace.   —*A Course in Miracles*

First Steps

Everyone is involved in the quest for healing. We live in toxic times, physically, mentally, and emotionally. Some of us experience a more urgent need for healing than do others, perhaps because an injury or illness has removed us from our comfortable (or uncomfortable) routines. Often our healing needs to occur at multiple levels—not just the body but the emotions and the mind as well.

When we begin a healing process, what do we anticipate? In the old days, a big part of getting well was expected to come from others. We could go to the doctor or other health practitioner, or perhaps a therapist or counselor, and let them take care of us. We might be given pills to take to feel better, or surgery, or a set of exercises to carry out.

Times are changing. Now, with the medical care system going through drastic upheaval, people are thrown much more onto their own resources. Gone are the days of prolonged hospital stays and multiple caregivers and therapies. This is both a blessing and a challenge. Many in the holistic health field have observed that the old medical establishment is crumbling as we move into an era of new thinking about the nature of health and illness.

More people are exploring both new and ancient ways of

healing, which are often not covered by their health insurance plans; they are investing in their health instead of in illness care. Americans now visit alternative medicine practitioners with greater frequency than physicians. Many are realizing that they can do a lot more of their own healing work themselves, with less reliance on professionals. Healing methods that rely on nature instead of technology, such as herbal medicine, are regaining popularity.

Taking so much responsibility for our own healing process is a bit scary, and we haven't been well prepared for it. Most of us were brought up to place our trust in medical professionals and to rely on them to take care of us, especially when we reach old age. Taking our power back can be both daunting and exciting. What I do now may determine whether or not I will even have an old age.

Healing involves mind, body, and spirit. Here are some of the steps I've found personally useful:

- Recognizing that I have a problem, and clarifying my intention to heal.
- Finding the support I need.
- Learning to honor and listen to my body and my inner guidance.
- Breathing and relaxation.
- Exploring ways to take care of myself.
- Working through emotions.
- Caring for the inner family.
- Releasing judgments and seeing in new ways.
- Letting go of victimhood.
- Living my dreams.
- Letting nature teach me and heal me.
- Creating community.

It's important to create a plan, including daily practices, and stick to it, revising it as necessary. Committing to a daily practice is like keeping an appointment with yourself. I have found that after about three weeks of any daily practice I've chosen, whether it's yoga, meditation, exercising, or singing, it starts to become natural, almost automatic. I'd miss it if I didn't do it. Sometimes if I've skipped a practice, I realize that my day isn't going nearly as well as it could have. At the same time, flexibility is essential for adapting to the ever-changing flow of life. A self-healing program must accommodate our fluctuating needs. Otherwise, a daily practice can become a chore or a "should." Each day offers many opportunities to wake up, many opportunities to laugh and to enjoy the gifts of the moment.

Intention

If you are certain, then you are a prisoner of the known.
When you embrace uncertainty, and include intention
and detachment, then the most improbable happens.
That's what we call a miracle. —Deepak Chopra, M.D.

Setting a conscious intention mobilizes our resources and power. As you begin any activity, remind yourself of your positive intention. You might want to state it aloud, write it down, and/or form a mental image of your goal. The clearer our intentions and the less conflicted we are, the more likely we are to get the desired result. Intention alone is not enough; we must add energy. I find that beginning my day with a clear intention has a powerful effect on the whole day.

The extent to which I open myself to receive from the universe determines what I'll get. Reminding myself, first thing in the morning, of a particular lesson from a favorite teacher, will activate that teaching for me later during the day. Gratitude or a small act of giving gets me off to a great start.

Tim Corcoran, who leads nature awareness classes in wilderness areas, often takes groups out for early morning walks and has them state what they would like to experience, such as, "I'd like to see a bear this morning," or "I want to experience the peace and beauty of nature today." Focusing on your intention to be well is a wonderful way to start your healing process.

I have a little set of "angel cards," and I often draw one before starting a morning meditation. Each card bears a tiny picture of an angel who embodies the quality printed on the card, such as forgiveness, generosity, humor, or flexibility. Focusing briefly on my angel card, I invite that quality to be present with me throughout the day. Angels are said to be messengers; perhaps they are invisible presences among us that whisper helpful words in our ears. But we have to ask for their help. If I call frequently enough on my angel of generosity, I can trust I'll be guided to be more generous without needing to plan it on a conscious level. The intention seems to have a life of its own, leaving me surprised at my willingness to give something away! On the other hand, one day when I had drawn the "honesty" angel I caught myself in a lie. The discomfort that ensued gave me a strong motivation to change my patterns.

One of my favorite ways to prepare myself with an intention of helpfulness in any situation is to state silently, "I am here only to be truly helpful." (The beginning of the "Healer's Prayer" in A Course in Miracles.)

Clear intention invites synchronicity: unlikely coincidences that are laden with meaning. A powerful intention is to open myself to guidance from any source that may come my way. For example, I was taking care of a baby who had a cold; as we came back from our walk, I saw a flower in a neighbor's yard that looked a lot like echinacea. Later that day I saw a picture of the same flower in a magazine. These encounters reminded me to take some echinacea extract to strengthen my immune system against the cold virus. I followed my guidance and didn't get sick.

One day I had a strong desire to find a certain passage in a 300-page book which a friend had recommended that I read. There were no clues in the table of contents. Much to my amazement, I had located the exact section I wanted within three minutes. Was this luck, synchronicity, or the result of intention?

It is helpful to have another person be a witness for an intention we want to bring forward. For example, a person who decides to quit smoking might announce this goal to a friend. Marriage always involves witnesses to the commitment made by the couple.

When we join our intentions with those of several other people, it is even more powerful. I once saw how a group's intention and focus helped a fire-maker, who was using a bow-drill, to succeed. For a while people's attention had strayed and just one man was working; finally he asked us all to focus our minds and help bring the fire into being. Within a minute, there was a burst of flame.

The purer the motive (the more it is free of ego), the greater the result. Form your intention, breathe energy into it, and then let it go. To bring your intentions into alignment with those of another person, or to establish rapport, begin to breathe with the person, matching your exhalations and inhalations.

Contrast the conscious intention with our society's usual "Type A" approach. In conscious intention, we intend, add energy, let go, and allow a result to occur. In the Type A approach, we intend, then we strive, take control, and try to force a result. There is no trust. Think of planting seeds. Once they are planted and watered regularly, and energized by the sun, there is nothing to do but allow the young plants to unfold. Digging them up to check on their progress only makes it more difficult for them.

Once I was on a camping weekend with a group, feeling frustrated with how difficult it had been to organize meaningful shared activities with so many people. The exciting possibility of having a dream-sharing session had been in my mind for a few days. I let go of trying to organize it, and began to tell my previous night's dream to just one person. Twenty minutes later, all nine of us were happily engaged in recounting our dreams to one another. My strong desire and intention to share dreams had resulted in a dream that was intriguing enough to spark everyone's interest; my enthusiasm for sharing it was sufficient to generate the intimate outpouring I had hoped for.

The intention and energy with which we speak or act makes a huge difference in the outcome. For example, a simple phrase, such as "I don't understand," may be uttered with angry, rejecting energy, or with loving intent and the desire to be closer. The intention behind the words often has more impact on the listener than the words themselves.

Exhale any time you are making an effort, and let go of unnecessary muscle tension. Intend for your goals to be accomplished effortlessly. To exhale helps us flow past obstacles; it is a form of releasing, letting go of trying, letting it be easy.

According to Brooke Medicine Eagle, a Native American teacher, we create results most powerfully by dancing and singing in a circle with focused intention. Through ceremony, and the power of the circle, we bring our energy into alignment with our intention; the outcome is much greater than hard work alone could produce.

I once spent a day with the conscious intention of wishing happiness for everyone I encountered. To my surprise, I felt more joyous and powerful than I could have imagined, despite the fact that there were many challenges going on in my life. Christiane Northrup, M.D., author of *Women's Bodies, Women's Wisdom,* suggests that we repeat to ourselves, nightly, for a month: "I'm intending vibrant health."

ASK YOURSELF: What are my strongest intentions for this day?

Finding Support

> *We're the first culture to create so much isolation for human beings. Now we are moving back toward community—because we need it to happen.*   —Gay Luce

Having support is a key aspect of the circle of healing. Have you ever watched two fish jump near each other in a pond? The concentric ripples fan out, like spheres of influence intersecting, overlapping, forming the infinity symbol, and finally converging into one larger circle. Sometimes I've chosen just one person to check in with about our progress toward our individual goals, and at other times I have started or joined a group. A support group can make a life-and-death difference among cancer patients, but why wait until we have a life-threatening illness? A great number of scientific studies show that social support is an essential aspect of healing. We all need some encouragement, a little nudge, or a bit of inspiration at times when the going gets tough.

What friend makes you laugh? With whom can you share your dreams, and plot how to make them real? Who gives you honest reality-checks? To whom do you turn when you're feeling low? With whom can you be your most un-edited self? It is rare that one person can provide all these supportive roles for us.

Humans are resistant to change, and we need to take this into account when we set out to do something new and challenging. How different it feels to walk into a roomful of strangers with a friend at your side, instead of by yourself. Support has many aspects. People move ahead faster when they hire the help they need to accomplish any goal, instead of berating themselves for not being able to do everything on their own. Often, as well, we can find a great deal of support for free—once we give ourselves permission to ask for it.

We all belong to families and have networks of friends who share some of the same patterns of behavior and habits we may want to change, and they can be a powerful force to reckon with. Anyone who has tried to quit smoking has probably experienced how difficult it is if one's friends continue to smoke. The puffing pals may even try to undermine their friend's resolve to kick the habit. Many times, our failure to reach a goal is not so much because we lack will power as because we lack the necessary social support.

I've also seen, and been in, support groups that actually kept people stuck in their old patterns. One group had an unspoken agreement that no one would challenge anyone else, and instead we took turns giving each other sympathy for how difficult it was to make any progress. If anyone had been successful, the other members would have felt envious. This was not a group that supported growth. Once I realized that my intention was not aligned with that of the group, I chose to leave it.

Just as a social group can be a force for resisting progress, it can also be a powerful boost toward making positive changes. The key is to find or create a group that will support you. For the would-be ex-smoker, the logical support group would consist of other people who are trying to quit, and/or nonsmoking friends who would love to help you reach your goal. If you notice that the group you are in is not helping its members in their stated goals, or if the culture of the group doesn't feel right to you, join or start another one.

Why and how do support groups work? Despite our cultural programming to be tough-minded "rugged individuals," we are truly social creatures. We fear being alone, isolated, different. When we are in pain (physical, emotional, or both), we are more vulnerable to such fears, and even more in need of support. And yet, at such times, our families and friends may be unable to understand what we are going through. They may feel afraid or inadequate. Often a support group will consist of people who are going through a similar challenge. Now, instead of feeling different, we are with people who share our experience. We can talk freely about our challenges and our weaknesses. This seems to unlock our innate desire to help one another, and can bring out the best in each person. Solidarity creates strength.

Ideally, people in support groups give us honest feedback. They provide a safe environment for taking a next step. They amplify energy in a wonderful way, making it possible for everyone to make progress. A healthy group nurtures the growth of its members and lets everyone be honest and real; instead of avoiding conflict, issues are brought out into the open. We don't have to solve all our own problems before we can help each other; by listening and offering empathy, our own difficulties seem to become smaller.

Other people also mirror us back to ourselves. When another

person has the same problem as I do, I can look into his or her eyes and see an aspect of myself that is suffering or in pain. In experiencing compassion for this person, it becomes easier to be compassionate toward myself. This phenomenon occurs regularly at the Center for Attitudinal Healing in Sausalito, California, an organization founded by Dr. Jerry Jampolsky. The Center's philosophy is that "we are all teachers and healers to one another." It began by offering peer support groups for children with life-threatening illnesses and now offers groups for the siblings of such children, for their parents, for children with seriously ill parents, and much more.

Years ago, a newspaper story about the Center for Attitudinal Healing made a deep impression on me. In a children's hospital room, a little boy whose right side was paralyzed lay in bed, depressed and withdrawn, not moving even his left arm. In a nearby crib, a baby with a brain tumor was crying. The little boy's mother, who had attended an Attitudinal Healing support group, picked up the crying baby with the assent of his mother. She placed the baby on the chest of her young son. Almost instinctively, the boy's left arm stroked the baby, who stopped crying. This moment marked the beginning of the paralyzed boy's recovery.

A similar philosophy is practiced by Patch Adams, the off-beat "funny doctor" made famous by the movie with his name. As a suicidally depressed young man in a mental hospital, Patch discovered that he was still able to help another patient, and this joyful experience lifted him out of his own mental illness. The desire to help others led him to attend medical school, and as a student he started a free clinic in which everyone (including the staff) is a patient, and everyone is also a healer.

Too often, people undergoing illness or emotional problems of any kind are placed in a position of powerlessness. We're steered toward therapists and social workers, people who make their living helping others. Not that these professionals aren't useful; they can indeed be extremely valuable and can save lives. However, our society differs from many others in our rather extreme reliance on paid professionals. This may be a symptom of how isolated we have become, how disconnected from true emotional closeness with others. How did people survive before Freud and psychotherapy (and all its spin-offs)? They talked to their minister or rabbi, their hairdresser, their extended family members, neighbors, work mates, and peers.

The sense of powerlessness that results from defining oneself as a patient or client generates a negative atmosphere for healing. Research on the immune system reveals a decrease in immune functions when a person feels helpless. In a study by Langer and Rodin, they found that the simple act of caring for a living plant, rather than having it watered by the staff, made a difference in the health of elderly nursing home patients.

As Rachel Naomi Remen, M.D., the medical director of the Commonweal Cancer Help Program, writes:

> We're all wounded. People who have lived life with any depth or taken any necessary risks in life have experienced loss and disappointment. The experience of being wounded, and what happens to one as one responds to the wound, gives us the wisdom to heal one another.

At Commonweal, cancer patients spend a week in a small group that attends classes and therapy groups, meditates, eats, and lives together. A deep feeling of closeness develops during that time. A friend of mine who went through the Commonweal program recalls how she was moved to tears when her group, who had decided to go howl at the full moon together one evening, insisted on including her and lovingly waited for her to complete a phone call.

Perhaps the most outstanding example of the transformative effect of social support is the breast cancer groups started by psychologist David Spiegel. Following surgery, the women who took part in these support groups, where they were able to discuss feelings with one another, lived twice as many months as a similar set of women who did not attend a group.

Another powerful force for change has been the "Twelve Step" groups, beginning with Alcoholics Anonymous and now including a group for nearly every addictive behavior including gambling and sex. These groups, which are led by peers and are financed only by voluntary donations, have been credited with assisting more people to full recovery than any other program or therapy.

Dean Ornish, M.D., who pioneered the first program to reverse heart disease without surgery, realized that a lowfat vegetarian diet, exercise, and stress management methods such as yoga and meditation were not enough. An integral part of his program is the support group. Indeed, he feels that most people would not be able to change their lifestyles so drastically if they were not part of a group going through a similar challenge. But most importantly, his program emphasizes "opening the heart," and that is what occurs when feelings are shared with a group of sympathetic people.

A support group need not be defined based upon a problem. It can also be a group with a common goal, such as learning to write; or a group with a common interest, such as creating rituals with their families, talking about their dreams, or discussing the ideas in a favorite magazine.

Many people are forming "simplicity circles" to discuss and implement ways to escape the rat race of materialism. The

NorthWest Earth Institute has helped thousands of people in the northwest, and now in many other regions as well, to start study circles on Voluntary Simplicity, Deep Ecology, Choices in Sustainable Living, and A Sense of Place. (See the "Resources" section at the end of this book.)

How can you get into a support group? There are groups for folks with a great variety of physical and emotional problems, from arthritis to chronic fatigue to widowhood. Check the phone book or the Internet. There is even a Self-Help Clearinghouse that can direct people into groups. (See "Resources.") There are free groups for people who want to explore career change, called "Wish Craft" groups (named for the popular book by Barbara Sher), which may be listed in your local paper. Free alternative weekly or monthly newspapers and magazines are a good source for such information. For those with access, the Internet can be a great resource.

One of the best ways to have a group that is tailored to your needs is to start one of your own. It may help to find one other person to start it with. That way leadership is shared from the outset. Many newspapers offer free classified ads for groups that do not charge a fee. To quote ChoQosh Au-Ho-Oh, a Native American elder, "Speak your truth and see who is drawn to you. Don't edit your heart. Be who you really are so your community can find you!"

A support group can become a wonderful source of friendships. I belonged to a group that studied and discussed A Course in Miracles and how it applied to our lives. We met weekly for about five years, and although the group no longer exists, the friendships continue. Over the years, I have participated in a variety of support groups, including a "Wish Craft" group, a grief support group, and several study circles based on the NorthWest Earth Institute's courses.

It's very nurturing to have someone to whom I'm accountable, who will be disappointed if I don't do something I've committed to and will cheer me on if I'm discouraged at my slow progress. Assisting another person's growth is a joyful and strengthening experience.

With one other person, I started a "Year to Live" group, based on the book with that title by Stephen Levine. We each called our friends, put out announcements on e-mail, and I placed an ad in the paper. One of the people who answered the ad, not knowing it was me, was an acquaintance I had not seen in several years! We chose to live one year as if it were our last, taking care of unfinished business and examining our most important priorities in life.

I'm currently in a group that began years ago with the purpose of acting on the ideas and world view expressed in the magazine *In Context*, whose successor is called *Yes! A Journal of Positive Futures*. We have done seasonal rituals, helped support one of our members who was diagnosed with cancer, assisted a member who was facing surgery, and now have a community garden.

HERE ARE SOME GUIDELINES FOR GROUPS:
1. An optimal size for a group is between four and ten people. Otherwise, the meetings may take too long, and/or some people may remain silent.
2. Sit in a circle if possible. Circles collect and focus energy, and give everyone equality.
3. Discuss the issue of keeping confidential what is shared within the group.
4. Make sure that each person has an opportunity to speak. Many groups pass a "talking stick" (or stone, or other

object) around the circle. The person holding it is free to
speak without being interrupted.

5. Be good listeners for one another, rather than advice-
givers. When someone is speaking, give full attention,
rather than planning what to say when it's your turn.

6. Create an atmosphere of nonjudgmental acceptance. Look
for the best in the other person. After all, whatever you
focus upon is what you give energy to. You might as well
focus on the person's highest expression, since that is the
aspect you wish to engage with. (Hint: Look for it in their
eyes.)

7. Speak from the heart, and listen from the heart.

A FINAL WORD ABOUT SUPPORT: You need not be in the same
room to experience the healing effects of loving intention. In a
remarkable study at San Francisco General Hospital, cardiac
patients who were prayed for were five times less likely to
require antibiotics, and three times less likely to develop pul-
monary edema, than a control group. These results occurred
despite the fact that neither the patients nor the doctors knew
which group was being prayed for, and the prayer groups knew
only the patients' names.

Have fun getting your support group started.

A Circle of Gifts

A community provides a safe space for people to open their
hearts and reveal who they are; it helps people to see, and
bring forward, their special talents. These gifts are then offered
back to the community, and everyone benefits.

A beautiful circle was done by our group on a member's
birthday. We each took turns speaking of her gifts, the special

qualities we saw in her and the ways we had received from her. Our modest friend blushed and glowed as she was acknowledged for her wonderful generosity, high ideals, community-building skills, and open-heartedness.

Later, at a time when I was feeling confused about my direction and starved for validation, the group spontaneously decided to do a "gift circle" for me. As each person spoke, my tears dripped onto the notebook in which I greedily tried to scribble down all their comments. What an experience of receiving pure love!

Dialogue

Honoring the Body's Wisdom

The body weeps the tears that the eyes refuse to shed.
—author unknown

Our culture has taught us to split the mind and the body, and to exalt the mind while assigning the body the inferior role. Many religious traditions depict the body as filled with desires, lust, laziness, and frailty. "The spirit is willing but the flesh is weak." The shaming of young children in toilet training reinforces this contempt for the body.

Suppose there was a servant living in your house. Although you clothed and fed him, you treated him with utter disdain. You barked orders at him, and never made eye contact. Assuming that he had nothing of value to say, you never listened to him. You treated him like a beast of burden, beating him just to remind him that you were the boss. There was no trust, for you accused him of laziness, greed, lust, and violence. Then suppose that this silent servant, whom you had abused for years, turned out to be the best friend you'd ever had. What if this long-enduring one was revealed as the wisest, most devoted and truthful ally, offering you the path to healing and wholeness?

Your body follows your orders faithfully. If you don't want it to feel, you will not be aware of feelings; but the emotions will be stored for you so that when you are ready, they can be experienced. When you open your mind and heart to yourself and listen attentively to your body, it dares to dream that you will honor its wisdom and wishes, that you will listen to its quiet protests. Slowly, trust is built, from one part of you (your mind) to the other part of you (your body).

It isn't really possible to separate mind from body; but if the illusion is there, a bridge of trust must be built. The body holds much wisdom and will share it if we are willing to listen. Our inner vulnerability speaks to us and communicates its hurts to us, through the body. In contrast to the constant chatter of the mind, the body's voice is quiet. Does your body have a communication for you? Would it be willing to answer a question you have?

The body never lies. We can say, "I'm not nervous," but our shaking hands and pounding heart tell another story. We learn to tune the body out when we don't want to hear the truth. Unacknowledged feelings may then show up as symptoms. If we try to medicate away the symptoms, they may recede for a while, only to show up in another form—still trying to get a message across.

When we reject that part that is hurting ("my bad back"), it's like whipping the servant who tries to speak. Many people disassociate themselves from a painful part of their bodies. Communication becomes more difficult, and healing is blocked. On the other hand, if we start to send love and respect to the body and to listen to its messages, communication begins to flow. Honor the messages received by acting on them appropriately, and slowly we can win back the trust of the disrespected and mistreated body. One of the greatest ways to practice self-acceptance and self-love is to honor the body and care for it. In my case, sometimes this means being patient enough to notice and release tension in my shoulders every half-hour.

Christiane Northrup, M.D., asks us: "How would your life be different if your body were your friend and ally, as valuable as a beloved friend or child? How would you treat yourself differently?"

The less rigidly we hold our bodies, the less rigidly we hold our beliefs and thoughts, and the more vigorously we live our lives. Relaxation helps us lighten up by letting go of what isn't working anymore. Practice deep relaxation every day if possible. Learn what it feels like to be awake yet fully relaxed in every muscle. Twenty minutes of deep relaxation once a day is a great way to start. Later you can give yourself a choice: twenty minutes once a day—or one minute, twenty times a day.

There are fascinating stories recounted in *The Heart's Code* by Dr. Paul Pearsall about heart-transplant patients who receive, along with the new heart, some of the likes, dislikes, and even memories of the donor. A prim and conservative elderly woman who received a young man's heart discovered a new fondness for beer and Chicken McNuggets. A young girl began having nightmares of murder after her heart transplant, with such vivid descriptions that they led to the identification of her donor's killer. Is it possible that every one of our organs, perhaps each cell, is filled with information and awareness? How can we tap the vast potential wisdom within our bodies?

As you develop the ability to be more present in your body and to live comfortably there, you'll develop more self-awareness and, with it, self-appreciation. As you come to know yourself better, you'll like yourself more. Our false ideas about ourselves generate self-rejection, which leads to pain, both emotional and physical. Stop shutting yourself out of your heart. Come home to your Self.

Begin to notice the ways in which your body is trying to communicate with you. Have you ever felt your gut ache when contemplating doing something you thought you "should" do but didn't want to? In the biofeedback clinic, clients have a literal opportunity to listen to their bodies' messages. Sensors are attached to the skin over a painful muscle group, and a signal can be displayed visually, while a sound will occur when muscle tension exceeds a set level. A client might say, "I don't think I'm stressed by my relationships at home," but their painful muscle "speaks up," registering an audible increase in tension!

One woman with an occupational arm-and-shoulder injury felt twinges of pain in her arms every time she talked about going back to work; her body was warning her not to become re-injured.

From Lucia Capacchione's books (*The Power of Your Other Hand* and *Recovery of Your Inner Child*), I learned a very simple way to have a dialogue with the body. It has helped me and it might work for you as well. The nondominant hand is connected to the hemisphere of the brain that is generally considered to be the intuitive part. Hold a pen or pencil with your dominant hand, and write down a question relating to an illness or problem you have. Then transfer the writing tool to your other hand and allow your intuitive self to express an answer. Writing with the nondominant hand can feel clumsy and slow, so give yourself as much time as you need. If you like, continue questioning with your dominant hand and answering with the other hand. At first this felt awkward and strange to me, but the more I've practiced it the more helpful it has become.

On a vacation trip, I realized that I had sustained several small injuries, all on the left side of my body: a scraped knee, a stubbed toe, a pulled muscle from kayaking, and a slight tear in the eardrum from diving. I took a pen in my right hand and asked what was going on. Then I took the pen in my left hand and wrote this message from my left leg: "Slow down. Even on vacation you try to do too much. That decreases your enjoyment. Have more quiet contemplation." Then my left arm suggested: "Don't overreach your limits." My left ear added: "Don't go too deep too fast." The overall message was: "Get into better balance."

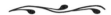

USING YOUR NONDOMINANT HAND, try completing this sentence: "When I hurt, my body is asking me for _attention_." If you prefer, use your nondominant hand to draw the answer to your question.

Communicating with Respect

In true listening, we reach behind the words, see through them, to find the person who is being revealed.
                                                     —John Powell

Positive relationships are founded upon certain principles of communication. The basic principles are the same, whether we are communicating between different parts of ourselves, between humans and animals, between family members, or between nations negotiating at the bargaining table. Communication involves listening and reflecting back what is heard, giving a message in a form which can be understood, listening for a response, and continuing until clarity is reached. The most important aspect of communication is respect, and respect means being willing to listen. Many people do not listen well, but merely take turns talking. Might this be because we live in such a noisy environment that we frequently need to practice selective listening? Or is it because we lack respect for the other, whether it is the other person, or an animal, or our own bodies?

Even a small error in communication can set off a nuclear war. Skillful communication, on the other hand, can establish a healing sense of connectedness with others, including not only other people but other life forms as well. Native Americans, along with great mystics like Saint Francis and Meister Eckhart, have referred to the sun, wind, water, trees, and animals as father, brother, sister— "All my relations." Many of us think of the earth as mother.

In fact, the prevalent modern sense of alienation and aloneness may spring from our disconnectedness from other people and from nature. As we lose the ability to connect and communicate in nonverbal ways with our multispecies extended family, human-to-human communication is impoverished. We rely on words and tend to neglect or ignore the many other ways in which communication is constantly occurring.

We have also forgotten how to listen within ourselves, to listen to the promptings and messages of our own bodies. If a symptom such as pain or illness signals us that something is out of balance, we can discover what is needed by attending to the message and learning how to translate it into a corrective action we can take. Rather than viewing the symptom as a nuisance that interferes with our plans, we can learn to value the body's messages, recognizing that they have information useful for our healing.

For some, the concept of having a dialogue with a symptom or a painful part of the body may seem odd. Wouldn't it be nice if we were so well in touch with our bodies' needs that no such communication was necessary? Unfortunately, we have learned to "tune out" the subtle messages of the body, so we must relearn how to listen in order to take better care of ourselves. The body's messages are an aspect of our intuition, our inner guidance system. I discuss this more in "What My Knee Knew." As we learn to relate better to our own bodies, we become able to relate better to nature, since our bodies are part of nature.

When I'm willing to take the time to communicate, I get the result I'm seeking: harmony. Great harmony, as in choral singing, requires time, listening, and patient practice.

Pay attention to the other's feelings and show that you heard those feelings. It isn't necessary to share in the feelings in order for empathy to be present, but it is necessary to refrain from judging the other. Notice your language. If you hear yourself contradicting another's point of view, using "but," "instead," or other words that oppose, try saying "and" or "or." Thus you put your alternative view alongside theirs, simply offering them an expanded array of choices.

Example:

A: "You said that to hurt me."

B: "But you weren't giving me any respect …"

Alternative:

A: "You said that to hurt me."

B: "Or I said it out of my own blindness and pain."

Most people are adept at disguising their beauty and greatness under a humble or abrasive exterior, designed to mislead us. We can only really see them if we are able to look past the facade. In any interaction with another, practice silently saying, "Namaste." The translation of this greeting is: "Spirit in me greets spirit in you." In this way we evoke the highest aspects of ourselves and others. Would we say, "The petty, critical nastiness in me salutes the self-centered stinginess in you"?

Whether you are seeking to communicate with a person, a symptom in your body, or another creature, many of the same principles hold true.

BASIC STEPS FOR COMMUNICATION:

1. Calm and center yourself, by taking a slow, deep breath and letting it out completely, a couple of times. Focus on letting go of tensions in your eyes, jaws, shoulders, belly. If you like, imagine putting roots down into the ground beneath you and letting any fear, anger, or other unwanted feelings be released into the ground. Imagine yourself standing inside a circle of safety. One of the biggest barriers to understanding one another is fear. As much as possible, speak from an open heart. Many people find it easier to open their hearts to a dog or cat than to another person. It doesn't matter where you start. The skill of open-hearted communication is transferrable.

2. Put aside judgments. Nothing closes down communication more surely than judgments, whether they be silent or spoken. What we want most from others is permission to be who we are! Describe the other's behavior in neutral language.

3. Practice respect. To respect means literally "to look again." Sometimes it is necessary to take a deeper look. It is easier for me to respect a child when I remember that each child has great potential, which is nurtured and fostered by the respect of adults. Respect means not giving unsolicited advice. Patience is a form of respect; it's giving time and space to those who are doing me the honor of communicating with me. If it is difficult to speak to someone with respect, it might help to practice focusing upon what you

admire or appreciate about this person.

4. Let go of any status difference; perceive the other as an equal, whether you are listening to your child, a caterpillar, or your aching back. Practice humility. Resonate with the other's point of view in any way that you can. In nature, an "I-Thou" relationship of subject to subject enables communication. If we commodify nature (seeing a tree as lumber), or in any way see the other as "less," we can't fully enter into relationship.

5. Listen more than you speak; seek to understand the other's viewpoint. Ask open-ended questions; allow for answers to come in unexpected ways, including nonverbal cues, movements, or gestures. Attend to your intuitions, and any feelings that come up. These are all part of listening. Sometimes, when I have a strong urge to interrupt, I've sent a thought-message instead. Although this is different from listening, it is often received surprisingly well.

6. Reflect back what you heard, especially any feelings or emotions being conveyed, to check for the accuracy of your understanding and to clear up any vagueness or uncertainty. Often we are unaware that we did not fully understand another's message. People love to know that they have been heard, even if the only way we can help is to convey our understanding. Giving an accurate acknowledgment of another person's viewpoint and feelings does not mean that you must agree. Acknowledging a child's feelings by saying, "I hear how angry you feel that you can't have a piece of candy now," can be more helpful than trying to distract her or telling her that candy isn't good for her.

7. Practice empathy. Marshall Rosenberg, author of *Nonviolent Communication*, suggests that we ask, "Are you feeling _____ because you're needing _____?"

This simple query lets people feel profoundly heard. It can work with symptoms too. Even if your guess is wrong, this question lets the other know that you care. They will be more open to sharing their emotions than if you simply ask, "How are you feeling?"

8. Honor the message by stating your response. If you are attempting to communicate with a headache, for example, and it is conveying a request for you to get more rest, decide whether or not you are willing to do that, and communicate your intentions. Stating intentions is equally important when communicating with people! If you are angry and need to take time out from an interchange, it might help to say, "I'm angry (or upset) right now and need to take a break to collect myself. I will get back to you in a half-hour."

9. Speak about your feelings rather than your intellectual judgments or defenses. Tell the truth without blame or judgment. There is a much better chance I will be heard when I say, "I feel hurt by the tone in which you said that," than when I say, "You're being rude." Also beware of "I feel that . . ." and "I feel like . . . ." These phrases are almost always followed by evaluations rather than emotions. The truth of our feelings is incontestable, but as soon as we begin to blame or criticize, the other party will shut down and become defensive. Communication comes to a halt.

10. Transform complaints into requests or suggestions. This allows the other to focus on meeting your request rather than defending against it. It also puts you in an empowered and creative position, rather than in a victim role. "It's too cold in here" becomes "Is it OK if I close this window?" Angeles Arrien tells a story of a tribal elder who, when given a chance to bring some problems to the attention of

government officials, did not bring up any complaints. His words were: "I regret that I have only three creative solutions to offer to solve these problems."

11. Instead of criticizing, appreciate. Look for the best in the other. Criticism rarely resolves problems; instead, it usually creates defensiveness and/or counterattacks. I heard about a day care center where a child who is angry or violent is simply held and comforted, perhaps even toted around for an hour or more, instead of being scolded.

If it is necessary to communicate negative feedback, it is much less stressful for both the communicator and the receiver to surround it with appreciation: An "appreciation sandwich" consists of a genuine statement of appreciation or acknowledgment, followed by the feedback, followed by another appreciation. For example: "I really appreciate your asking me if this is a good time to talk. The issue I want to bring up with you is that last night I was bothered by your comment about my weight. I realize that you are genuinely concerned with my health." A request might be added, such as, "I would like you not to discuss my weight with other people."

When communicating with a symptom in the body, we can appreciate it for any benefits it has conferred, such as time off from work, or an opportunity for reflection. Also, appreciate all the parts of yourself that are healthy. This practice invites more health. Appreciation is a form of love that is vastly underutilized. Researchers at the University of Washington have discovered that couples who stay together tend to have five times more positive interactions than negative ones. Child development researchers Betty Hart and Todd Risley found that children who were the most intelligent, self-confident, and flexible at age six had

received five times more positive than negative inter-
changes with their parents. That's a pretty good ratio to
give to ourselves, as well.

12. Keep your agreements. If you commit to taking an action,
be sure to follow through with it. Otherwise, you are breaking your word. It is easy to promise your cat you will spend
more time playing together and then to forget all about it.
When you are dialoguing with a symptomatic part of yourself, it is very important to stick to any agreements you
make. Too often, after a symptom disappears, we tend to go
back to our old habits. Keep your word to animals and
symptoms as much as you would to people. If you find that
it is not possible to keep an agreement, renegotiate until
you have a new plan that is mutually satisfactory.

AN EXCELLENT BOOK ON COMMUNICATION is Marshall
Rosenberg's *Nonviolent Communication: A Language of
Compassion*. For more ideas on how to dialogue with a
symptom, I highly recommend *Healing Yourself* by Martin
Rossman, M.D., and *Creating Wholeness* by Peper and Holt.
To learn communication with animals, Penelope Smith's *Ani-
mal Talk* is an excellent primer.

Relaxation: Inviting Images

Relaxation has many benefits for health. As chronically
tense muscles release, blood pressure decreases and restorative
body processes take place, including improved digestion and
enhancement of the immune system. Many illnesses have a
stress-related component, or become worse under stress. The
practice of relaxation also relieves anxiety. Contracted muscles

close us down mentally, emotionally, and spiritually, while relaxation opens us up.

Deep relaxation also offers access to the mind's fascinating storehouse of information. When the muscles are quiet, the conscious rational left brain drops some of its defenses, allowing access to intuition in the form of images, words, and thoughts, which arise spontaneously.

For some people, simply lying down results in falling asleep immediately. It may help to sit in a chair while doing imagery exploration. A few slow deep breaths may be sufficient to enter a deeply relaxed yet alert state of mind.

For others, muscle tension and a jumble of thoughts may make relaxation challenging. A relaxation tape, either purchased or recorded yourself from the following script, will be beneficial. If you decide to make your own tape, be sure to speak slowly and calmly, and pause for a few seconds between phrases. (You may purchase one of the author's relaxation tapes by using the order form or calling the 800 number at the back of this book.)

Be sure that you will not be disturbed while relaxing: Unplug the telephone, hang a sign on the door, negotiate with family members. Earphones can help minimize outside noise. Loosen your belt, remove eyeglasses, empty your bladder, get comfortable. Place a pad of paper and pen, pencil, markers or crayons nearby.

Sit or lie down comfortably. Close your eyes and slowly scan your body . . . . Take an easy, deep breath and as you let it go, release any tension in your jaw . . . . Allow your tongue to be cradled in your mouth . . . . Let your eyelids relax . . . . How much can you release the tension behind your eyes? . . . How much can you soften the skin over your temples? . . . Bring your awareness to your shoulders . . . . Release and let go of any tension . . . . Breathe comfortably . . . . Allow relaxation to flow like a warm wave, down your shoulders and arms, right out to the tips of your fingers . . . . Feel your body relaxing . . . .

Bring your awareness to your neck and invite it to release any tension . . . . Let a warm wave of relaxation flow down your spine to your shoulder blades, loosening and releasing . . . . With each comfortable breath, your spine becomes more supple and relaxed . . . midback . . . and lower back . . . very relaxed . . . . Bring your awareness to your chest, and feel the slow, steady pulsation of your heartbeat . . . lungs opening to receive the gift of breath . . . . Feel your abdominal muscles relaxed and soft . . . belly rising and falling effortlessly with the breath . . . all inner organs calm and comfortable . . . pelvis relaxed . . . . Feel how relaxed your whole upper body is becoming . . . . Surrender to wave upon wave of relaxation, cleansing your body of all tension . . . .

Relax your buttocks . . . legs . . . thighs . . . knees . . . calves . . . and feet . . . . Imagine that you can exhale tension out through the soles of your feet . . . . Letting go more and more with each breath . . . . Let the river of your breath flow through your entire body, unchanneled . . . . Imagine yourself at the top of a flight of stairs, going down so effortlessly it's like floating . . . . Ten, nine, eight . . . with each descending step, becoming more and more comfortably relaxed . . . . Seven, six, five . . . going into a deeply relaxed state of mind . . . . Four, three . . . deeper and deeper . . . two, and one.

Now find yourself in a place in nature, which is beautiful, safe, peaceful, and serene . . . . Feel the warmth of the sun on your body . . . . Notice what season it is, and what time of day . . . . Hear the sounds . . . and observe the colors and textures of all that surrounds you . . . . Feel the ground under your feet . . . . Take some time exploring this lovely spot, and making yourself at home in it . . . . Breathe in the fresh sweetness of the air . . . .

Bring to mind the area of your health that concerns you . . . .
Just look and feel inside to notice what this area is like at this
moment in time . . . . Allow any image, sensation, or thought to
occur. There may be a picture, a bodily sensation, a word or
phrase, or an emotion . . . . Whatever occurs, let it be . . . .
Observe from all angles, noting every detail . . . color, shape, size
. . . feeling tone . . . warmth or coolness . . . lightness or heaviness
. . . . Does it have a message to communicate to you? You might
ask it what it wants to say . . . or what it needs from you . . . and
allow time for a response, which may come in words or in pictures or feelings . . . . Ask it another question if you wish, or if
the first response was not clear . . . . Take your time . . . . Thank
it for whatever it has conveyed to you now, and let go of the
image . . . .

Imagine yourself beginning to fill up with healing light . . . .
Feel the healing taking place . . . bringing complete health and
wholeness . . . and allow it to continue . . . . Congratulate yourself for enhancing your health . . . . Know that the healing
process goes on at all times, beneath our awareness . . . .

And when you feel that this process is complete . . . return
briefly to your natural place of peace and serenity . . . which is
always there waiting for you to visit . . . . Take your leave, and
begin ascending the staircase to come back to fully awake consciousness . . . . One, two, three . . . coming up slowly . . . . Four,
five, six . . . feeling refreshed . . . . Seven, eight . . . with full awareness of the messages received . . . . Nine, and ten. Eyes open,
alert and feeling better than before.

NOW TAKE A FEW MOMENTS to write about your image, and
perhaps to draw it. Do this right away while it is still fresh in
your mind. Like dreams, these images often fade rapidly from
awareness.

For relaxation tapes, please see the "Resources" section at
the end of this book.

What My Knee Knew

One of my personal patterns has been to refuse to acknowledge some of my feelings, and then to develop a physical
symptom. My body does its best to get a message across to me
so that I will deal with the emotional issue. Symptoms are
part of my intuitive guidance system, pushing me to make
changes. Sometimes a symptom is an ingenious metaphor or
pun. If my face is broken out in blemishes, I might ask, "What
is it I need to *face*? What's asking to be *cleared up*?" I have
learned to listen by using the technique of left-hand writing
(described in "Honoring Your Body's Wisdom") and also by
inviting images to come and communicate with me while I'm
in a state of deep relaxation.

An image may not seem to make sense at first, but if we stay
with it and ask questions, its meaning usually becomes quite
clear. The more we practice opening up to our images, the
more easily we receive information.

My left knee began to bother me for no apparent reason. I
had not experienced any injury; it just hurt and felt weak when
I was walking up or down a hill. Then one day after I'd walked
a lot, it hurt so much that I started to limp, and I knew it was
time to check in and find out what was going on.

I closed my eyes, relaxed deeply, and invited an image for the
problem to come into my mind. I didn't see much except two
rigid lines looking like tight muscles outside my knee. When I
asked the image what the problem was, I was amazed at the
answer. My knee said, "You're doing too much, moving too

fast. Walk, don't jog. Slow down, be more patient and demand less of yourself." Looking back at myself from the point of view of my knee, I appeared quite driven, even though I was under the delusion that I was living a rather laid-back existence. I did realize that in fact, I was moving too quickly into a new relationship without having had time to recover from the previous one; I was looking for a new place to live; and I was pressuring myself to write this book.

With my right hand I wrote, "What are you trying to tell me, left knee?" With my left hand I answered, "Fear of going up and down, emotional highs and lows. Fear of emotional intensity and risk. Imbalance." So, I made an agreement with my knee to slow down and do one thing at a time, and not to rush into relationships.

The second time I invited an image of my knee to appear, I saw a large black ball, which at first looked like a cannon ball; then it might have been a bowling ball, and finally a ball and chain. The cannon ball was shooting out at great speed. Was the image telling me I was a "loose cannon?" Again I was being told that I was moving too fast. The bowling ball seemed to represent the possibility of just rolling along and having fun. But the image that had the most power for me was the ball and chain. When I questioned it, the ball and chain told me it was locking me up and grounding me because I wasn't setting clear enough limits. It asked that I restrict my own freedom a little and establish stronger boundaries so it wouldn't have to do that for me.

Afterwards I sat down to write about how I could better honor my boundaries. I decided to take no one's advice without determining that it fit. Instead of retreating into the safety of my thoughts, I would acknowledge the places where I felt fearful and avoid going into overdrive in an effort to push through. I committed to breathe and ground myself, to step back from my tendency to overreact, and to look at choices.

On another level, I started looking at how I walked. People had often told me that I dragged my left leg a little, with a stiff knee. So I started to bend my knee more and pick up my feet as I walked, as if stepping over something. "Don't 'trip'!" I said to myself, and imagined that I was stepping over obstacles and difficulties with each mindful step. Also, I noticed occasionally that I was landing harder on my left foot than my right. When I paid attention, I could walk more lightly, with a greater sense of balance, which was a very pleasant experience. I began doing calf stretches and swimming more. Meanwhile, my doctor sent me to a physical therapist, who gave me some strengthening exercises to do. By the time I saw the therapist, the problem felt nearly resolved, although I did the exercises and noticed continued improvements.

You may wonder how well I kept my agreements with myself about slowing down, grounding, and setting limits. One aspect of feeling more grounded for me is to spend more time in nature, and I make sure to do that. I jog less and walk a lot more. The new relationship I was rushing into came to an end because of doubts and unreadiness on both sides. As a result, my life simplified considerably. I learned a valuable, if painful, lesson about how not to end and begin relationships. Perhaps my knee was the messenger chosen by my deeper mind to communicate this lesson to the rest of me.

The Inner Guide

*The ability to draw consciously upon your nonphysical
guidance and assistance, to communicate consciously with
a nonphysical Teacher, is a treasure that can not be
described, a treasure beyond words and value.*

—Gary Zukav

A wonderful way to get in touch with the wisdom within is through the help of an inner guide. Martin Rossman, M.D., in his book *Healing Yourself,* recommends calling upon an "inner advisor," and notes that it can take any form the imagination supplies. Many people believe that we each have several guides, which can be animal, human, or angelic in form.

In some shamanic traditions, each person has a helpful and protective "power animal" that can be called upon at times of need or confusion. Anthropologist Michael Harner teaches people to find the power animal by means of a special inward journey, led by the sound of drumbeats, down an imaginary tunnel into the "underworld." Whatever animal, bird, or reptile of friendly aspect is seen four times is the power animal, and can be brought back for oneself (or for another person). Beginning when I was about seven years old, I was fascinated with deer and collected little ceramic deer figures; I read *Bambi* eight times. Years later when a partner did a shamanic journey for me, I was not surprised that a deer was my power animal.

Do these guides exist outside our own imagination? I leave that to you to decide. My belief is that all beings on the physical and spirit levels are deeply joined.

Our intuitive guidance emerges most easily under certain conditions. The drumming used in the shamanic journey is believed to give access to that realm by entraining the brain waves into a slower, theta rhythm. Theta waves have long been associated with greater flow of spontaneous imagery, as well as creativity. Biofeedback researchers Elmer and Elyse Green used EEG feedback to train people to shift into theta waves; after these sessions, people often reported arriving at spontaneous solutions to problems. The dream-like theta state can also be reached through deep relaxation, although we may move quickly through it into sleep.

Once deeply relaxed, you need only to set your intention: Invite a guide to join you, taking any form (human, animal, or angelic). Then allow whatever comes. You can discuss any question or problem with your guide, who may communicate to you in words or symbolic images. Consulting my inner guide allows me to let go of having to make every decision myself. What a comfort!

Sometimes guidance comes in dreams, especially when we ask a direct question before going to bed. When I had a cold that wasn't going away, I asked for a message in a dream. The next morning I had my answer: Fast from all food for one day. I followed this directive, and by the end of the following day my symptoms had disappeared.

My own favorite guide is Saint Francis, who seems to prefer being called "Francesco" or "beloved brother" more than "saint." Not having been raised Catholic, I was astonished at how profoundly moved I was by the movie *Brother Sun, Sister Moon*, which is about Francis' early life. The first time I saw it, I knew I had just had a life-changing experience; I remember the tears still flowing down my face as I rode my bicycle home. So many teachings jumped out at me from that film, that even after watching it ten times or more I still receive something new. The great popularity of this saint may be because he was not born one; he died to his ego-self and was reborn into Spirit. In the film this rebirth is depicted in a scene where Francesco is drawn outdoors from his sickbed by the tiny bird chirping on the windowsill, and holds it lovingly in his hands. Before he was seen as a spiritual leader, most people thought he was crazy. That gives us permission to be "crazy on our way to sainthood."

As I read and learned more about Francesco's deep connection with nature and all of creation, my admiration and love grew. At moments when I sought direction, he began to speak to me. It was also his influence that led me to nature for guidance.

A few years ago, I was doing an imagery session on my own to gain insight on how to treat uterine fibroids for which I had been receiving acupuncture. At first, I seemed to see Francesco, then he disappeared. I felt disappointed. Then, as if from very far away, I heard a voice calling: "Flavonoids! Flavonoids!" I didn't know what flavonoids were, but I reported this communication to my acupuncturist a few days later. His eyes got very round and without a word, he dashed into the other room to get his book of herbal remedies. Pointing to an entry, he said, "I was just planning to put you on this new herbal mixture, which contains bioflavonoids!" I wish I could say that the fibroids promptly went away, but many imagery sessions and many herbs later, I am coexisting peacefully with them to this day. After having a dream in which my fibroids were the elbow of a baby about to be born, I began to see them as a reminder of my unexpressed creativity. They have been faithfully prompting me to write this book.

In another encounter with Francesco, this time concerning my work, a scene from *Brother Sun, Sister Moon* flashed into my mind. It was a scene where he singlemindedly, almost fanatically, focuses on gathering stones for the rebuilding of the little San Damiano church. I asked him about this and was told that I needed to narrow my focus and do fewer things, rather than scattering my energies. He exemplified living in true simplicity, asking, "Why should we not live as the birds? They need only a few berries and a sip of water."

Francesco has taught me a lot about when to say "No." There is a scene in that film depicting the young Francesco, recently recovered from his illness, sweating and suffering in the unnatural atmosphere of the church his parents attend. Suddenly he cries, "No!" and runs out into the clear air, bright sun, and beauty of the spring countryside, where the divine spirit is so much more present for him. One day when I was doing what others expected of me but feeling miserable because I knew it was not my true work, that scene came back to me as a sweet reminder of the need to say "No!" to what is not life-affirming. Francesco admonished me to stop all joyless work, and go to wild places.

In a dream, some people were gazing at a painting representing Saint Francis. The canvas was a rich brown, with faint sketches of many animals and other life forms in it. Superimposed on this background was a green outline of a small man with outstretched arms, both embracing and including all of life. "Imagine," I said to the others, "the power of being able to communicate with all species—yet such humility!"

Breath: the Gateway

Conscious Breathing

Go slowly. Breathe and smile.   —Thich Nhat Hanh

Our breath is one of the most amazing aspects of being alive. The flow of breath is the movement of spirit through matter. In many spiritual traditions, breath is much more than exchange of oxygen and carbon dioxide: It is connection with life force. "Inspiration" refers not only to breathing, but to being filled with spirit or insight. Most of the time we breathe unconsciously, unaware of the quality or the depth of each breath. In today's world, most people breathe quickly and shallowly in the upper chest. Such a restricted breathing pattern is not only a result of anxiety, but also a contributor to stress and poor health. By simply paying attention to our breath, we can experience a wonderful integration of body, mind, and spirit. Nothing can bring us back to the present moment more effectively than awareness of our breathing.

Our breath is a metaphor for how we live. Our society puts more emphasis on the inbreath than the outbreath: more on achieving, striving, and filling up than on releasing and letting go. Notice whether you tend to breathe in again before your exhalation is completely finished. A healthy breathing pattern is to exhale twice as long as we inhale, with a slight pause at the end of the exhalation.

Start to explore your breathing patterns. If at any time you feel light-headed, nervous, or uncomfortable, it could be because you are breathing too fast. Prolong the exhalation by pursing your lips and letting the air out very slowly, perhaps taking as much as eight or ten seconds to exhale. Allow a comfortable pause at the end of the exhalation. This is also an excellent remedy for panic attacks. If you ever feel so frightened that it seems just impossible to breathe, try tightening up your body even more; then suddenly release the tension. After this you will probably be able to breathe more freely.

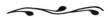

PRACTICES TO DEVELOP CONSCIOUS BREATHING:

1. To discover the natural way of breathing, observe a sleeping cat or dog. With each inhalation, the belly expands outward, and with each exhalation, the belly flattens. This is diaphragmatic breathing, and it is the most natural and relaxing way to breathe. Imitate the animal.

2. Breathe gently and lovingly into your whole body. Begin by breathing consciously while lying on your back. Place your hand on your abdomen, and let the breath move to meet your hand. Exhale fully, feeling your belly flatten, and allow yourself to let go of unwanted tensions, pain, and emotional upsets. Notice where in your body the exhalation seems to complete itself.

3. Sit up and practice breathing this way, with your hand on your abdomen: Inhale and expand; exhale and contract. Letting your spine be erect allows your breath to flow more easily through your body.

4. Breathe consciously as you start your day: Take five slow, deep breaths before getting out of bed.

5. Breathe and stand in the sun, taking in its energy, warmth, and light. Whenever we breathe consciously, we are inviting more life force energy into our lives.

6. Breathe with awareness while doing simple activities (such as walking, showering, or washing dishes). Be especially aware of your exhalations. Are they completed before the next breath begins? Can you keep your breath flowing without holding it, as you exert yourself?

7. Breathe consciously, whenever you remember, throughout the day. One minute a day. One minute, twice a day. Five minutes a day. We are usually distracted by too many stimuli (traffic, music, scenery, talk, thoughts) to be aware of our breath. Take steps to decrease the complexity of life, whenever possible, so as to make room for the simple and most important things, like breathing.

8. Breathe consciously through the little stressors. Relax your belly and reassure yourself.

9. Breathe with awareness through the big stressors.

10. Breathe consciously whenever you remember, and notice how much more spaciousness breath brings into your life.

Breath and Energy

Listen, are you breathing just a little, and calling it a life?
—Mary Oliver

Sickness or pain may result from an unskillful handling of energy: Sometimes we shut down our energy because we don't know how to handle it or we're afraid it may lead to pain. We may tighten up or clench because we believe we have to be "tough" to get through something. By shutting down our sensitivity and pushing our way through, we hurt ourselves and stress our system; injury or illness may result. To heal, we need to reconnect with our life energy.

"Breathing is the link between the mind and the emotions in the body," says Dan Millman, author of *The Way of the Peaceful Warrior.* "Bringing the breath back into balance helps bring our life back into balance."

Once I was on a backpacking trip and I wasn't feeling strong enough to carry my heavy pack. I didn't want to appear weak to my partner by asking for help with my load, so I clenched my teeth and tightened my belly in my attempt to be tough. At the end of the day I had quite a stomach-ache! A more skillful approach would have been to form a conscious intention to reach my destination and channel the necessary energy into carrying it out—and to ask for help if needed.

Sometimes we unconsciously make a choice to shut down our energy because having "too much" energy scares us—we feel uncentered and ungrounded. This leads to addictive behavior like drinking or overeating, or compulsively over-working—whatever it takes to feel numb. At such times, if possible, go for a brisk walk, breathe deeply, and feel how your energy allows your body to move. Or, imagine breathing in and out through your feet or your toes. Bring your awareness into your legs and feet. Picture yourself as a tree with roots firmly established deep in the ground. With each inhalation, draw energy up through your roots, feeling your connection with the Earth, letting yourself be nurtured and sustained. With each exhalation, release and let go of any energy you do not want, sending it back down into the vast Earth, which easily disperses and neutralizes it or puts it to another use. Exhale whenever you are startled, anxious, or angry. Breathe out your pain or resentment.

In Victorian times, when women wore corsets, frequent fainting was considered normal. Smelling salts and "fainting couches" were in widespread use. These women couldn't breathe! When I was a teenager, girdles were all the rage. Even now, when women are supposedly liberated, many are terrified of having bellies and automatically hold their abdominals tight, making healthy breathing impossible.

Often we don't breathe deeply because we learned early in life that we were not supposed to take up too much space, that we mustn't be too energetic. Many parents become annoyed when children make noise, won't sit still, jump around, and make demands. As a result, we learn to pacify ourselves and lower our energy level. One way to do this is with food. Overeating damps down our energy, while letting the defiant rebel in us take up more space. Excess weight adds a layer of protection between our vulnerable energy center and the world. When you feel like overeating, try breathing deep in your abdomen and reassuring yourself that it is fine to take up as much space as you want. Welcome your own energy and utilize it to accomplish your goals, or release it harmlessly.

I've noticed my tendency to eat when I have too much nervous energy and am trying to calm myself down. It has nothing to do with being hungry. At those times I need to stop and ask myself, "Why am I nervous and what is making it hard for me to settle down? What needs to be expressed?" Simply admitting to myself the reasons I am jittery goes a long way toward making me calmer.

We can choose to increase our life force energy at any time, by breathing more deeply and exhaling more completely. A change in the body sends a different message to the mind. We teach our minds through our behavior. Taking slow, deep breaths in the midst of a conflictual situation sends a message to our inner core that there is nothing to fear, thus allowing the mind to calm down. In the biofeedback clinic, where a number of physiological responses can be monitored and displayed, it is remarkable to observe how the skin conductance response (the sweat on our fingers when we are stressed) can decrease dramatically with slower breathing.

In times of intense feelings, breathing fully has helped me to sail through and emerge on the other side of a difficult emotion. It reminds me of a car approaching a large mud-puddle. If I put on the brakes as I hit the puddle, I might be stuck in there for a long time. If I step on the accelerator a bit, my car will get wet and muddy, but is less likely to stall in the middle.

Breathing deeply enhances receptivity. To breathe consciously, while experiencing an emotion, doesn't decrease the intensity of the emotion; it may even increase it. The breathing allows you to expand around the emotion and let it flow through you, while realizing that you are bigger than the emotion. Thus breathing deeply gives you an alternative to:

- feeling completely taken over by the emotion;
- getting stuck in the emotion;
- suppressing the feeling or only partly feeling it.

ASK YOURSELF THROUGHOUT THE DAY, if you observe your energy diminishing, "What am I making more important than my aliveness?" Then choose again. When you feel stuck, breathing deeply will help you discover your feelings. You might want to write or talk about your feelings, or draw them.

Exhale away any negativity you experience around you. Push it away with your breath—aggressively, if you like. Go ahead, pretend all the negativity is "out there." It doesn't matter, because as you exhale, you can let go of the inner negativity as well. Consciously exhale completely through your mouth, and as you do, picture all the stuff you don't want in your space flowing far, far away from you, dispersing and dissolving.

Whenever your breath shuts down, your jaw clenches, or your shoulders tighten, try asking yourself:

- Am I forgetting to breathe? (Take a deep breath.)
- What am I afraid of at this moment? (Name the fear.)
- What would a courageous person do now? (Picture it.)

Lighten Up!

> *He who binds to himself a Joy*
> *Does the winged life destroy.*
> *But he who kisses the Joy as it flies*
> *Lives in Eternity's sun rise.*
>
> —William Blake

To lighten up, stop being hard on yourself. Don't be the "heavy."

When you don't understand, laugh! Let the rascally side of you come out and play.

Put more air in your body: Breathe deeper to get lighter.

What could you do more lightly in your life?

Lighten up your attitude.

Lighten up your spirits.

Lighten up your judgments of yourself.

Lighten up your touch.

Lighten up your diet (less meat and dairy, more fruits and veggies).

Lighten up your walk.

Lighten up your grip on the steering wheel.

Lighten up your touch on the keyboard.

Lighten up your speech (suggest instead of insist).

Lighten your load by shedding possessions and obsessions!

Live lightly: Leave a smaller footprint on the Earth.

Lightly: gently, delicately, with little weight or pressure, buoy-
antly, without emotional heaviness, quietly, easily, nimbly,
without effort or intensity, humorously, cheerfully, with a
carefree spirit.

Levity is the opposite of gravity. What does weightlessness
mean to you? When was a time you felt truly light on your
feet? To learn about lightness, hang out with a butterfly.
Observe all the winged ones. Flying insects, birds, angels—
they are all in cahoots!

Lightness above me, lightness below me, lightness in front of
me, lightness behind me, lightness to my left, lightness to my
right, lightness inside me, lightness all around me.

Breathe in the light. Breathe out the light.

> *The angels fly because they take themselves lightly.*
>
> —G. K. Chesterton

Healing

Choices

*If each of us were involved in some form of positive
change, there wouldn't be enough problems to go around.*
—Sam Harris

Life is about choosing priorities. To give your body's
innate healing system a big boost, put a high priority on
doing what you love. Choose joy. As you do the things
that feel natural and wonderful to you, you invite a flow of positive energy powerful enough to overcome the energetic block-
ages that create illness.

Here's a list of suggestions to help you in your healing
process. Pick one or two that appeal to you and start there.
Give yourself lots of choices—no more shoulds and have to's.
Having choices moves you out of victim status. Remember
that taking a very small step toward healing is far better than
doing nothing. It starts the process; it mobilizes the part of you
that wants to heal; and the next step will be easier.

Ask yourself: "In what ways am I under stress?" Be sure to
take into account the stress of newness. Any change in routine, even if it is a positive change, involves letting go of the
old. Just acknowledging that change is difficult can help.

If you're afraid of change, feel the fear, breathe deeply, and
start with the most *fun* thing (not necessarily the safest). Pick

what makes you feel most alive. Then, congratulate yourself. Gradually you'll find yourself more and more willing to tackle the tough areas, such as the addictions, and you'll find your attachment to old habits lessening as your life becomes juicier. Stop criticizing yourself in any way. Start complimenting and acknowledging yourself for everything positive you do. Speak gently and positively to yourself, as though you were speaking to an anxious child. Or, if you like, congratulate yourself outrageously! Brag to the mirror until you laugh. My youngest brother, Michael, introduced me to a practice he invented for himself, which he called his "Yeas":

> I think of my goals, like around my music, my band, and I say "yea" to myself for anything I did yesterday that helped me reach my goals. Those are my "band yeas." I also have "food yeas" when I eat healthier.

I was very impressed by this simple practice of self-love, and began spending time acknowledging myself every day, even for the smallest things: "I am pleased with myself for saying no when I didn't want to go out, even though it would have been easier to say yes." It helps me to acknowledge myself for attitudinal changes as well as for accomplishing tasks.

Find enjoyable ways to exercise, such as walking in beautiful places, dancing, riding a bicycle, swimming—whatever you like best. Physical movement helps the process of inner movement and change of every kind. It's more than a metaphor for overcoming inertia and mobilizing health. Movement causes our blood to circulate vigorously, carrying healing into all parts of our bodies. It causes a cascade of endorphins, which produce a natural high and a delicious boost in self-esteem as well. Exercise is the single most powerful depression-chaser.

Spend time outdoors daily. The more natural the setting, the better. Our bodies were evolved to spend time in nature, not indoors with stale air and artificial lighting. Why walk on a treadmill or sit on a stationary bike in a gym, going nowhere, when you could be enjoying trees, birds, flowers, and passers-by? Warren Grossman, author of *To Be Healed by the Earth*, says: "Health is not possible without daily outdoor activity. . . . Only outdoor exercise moves enough of the Earth's energy through the body to strengthen and support it sufficiently for the work of life."

Send love, often, to whatever within you hurts or is unwell. Send a smile to it.

Spend one-on-one time connecting deeply with a friend or loved one. Hang out with people you like, respect, and learn from—especially friends who make you laugh.

Drink extra water for purification and cleansing within.

Do things that are positive for the planet. We depend on a clean environment for health. The Earth's health is our health.

Be kind. Anonymous acts of kindness are powerfully life-affirming. Here are some of my favorites:

• Silently send a wish for well-being and happiness to another person, or to several people. (It takes only a few seconds.)
• Pick up some trash from a park, or a sidewalk. (Imagine if everyone did that.)
• Smile at a stranger (kids are the most fun!)

When you feel down, depressed, in pain: give to yourself. Often our tendency is to judge and punish ourselves at such times. Do something you love to do, whatever it is, as long as it's not a compulsive, numbing-out behavior such as eating, drinking, smoking, drugs, TV, overworking. You know which ones these are for you. When I feel down, sometimes I ask myself what would nurture me most. This has prevented me

more than once from thinking I have to "compensate" myself
with chocolate.

Even when you're not depressed, do something that gives
you joy, daily. It's good preventive medicine. Keep a list handy
of all the healthy pleasures you enjoy; for instance:

- Go for a walk (especially at the beach or in the woods).
- Take a bike ride.
- Draw or paint.
- Listen to, sing, or play music, or sing along with your favorite
  music.
- Read inspirational writings, or humor.
- Listen to a relaxation tape.
- Give yourself a little massage (or get one from a friend).
- Dig in the garden.
- Take a hot bath with scented oil, or bubble bath.
- Light incense and/or candles.
- Talk to or write to a friend.
- Write in your journal.
- Dance.
- Bounce and shake out your arms and legs.
- Tell a joke to a friend and laugh.
- Play a game.
- Feed the birds.
- See an uplifting and/or humorous movie (or video). Try
  Groundhog Day.
- Rise to the occasion. Walking with a friend, we encountered
  a crying child holding onto a fence while his mother gently
  tried to persuade him to let go. My impulse was to smile sym-
  pathetically in her direction and keep going. But my friend
  stopped in her tracks and looked, as if astonished, at the
  child. He looked back with curiosity and stopped crying.
  Then she began walking a very silly walk, making faces all

the while; the child watched silently. In a moment he was walking calmly with his mother. Afterwards, my friend confided: "I asked myself, 'What would Patch Adams do here?'"

* Take a monthly "fast" day (fasting from food, driving, e-mail, or the news) The amazing thing about *fasting* is that it causes us to *slow down*. One day a month spent fasting in a natural place works like a mini-Vision Quest, clearing my mind and attuning me with nature.

* Perform experiments. For example, try going off dairy products or sugar for a week or two, long enough to observe whether your experiment has made a positive difference. If you like the results, continue; if not, don't.

* Borrow a friend's kid for a few hours if yours are grown or you haven't any.

* Sing your own song, whatever it may be. Honor your own uniqueness by giving expression to it. When we're singing our own song, we don't have any missing notes.

AT THE END OF THE DAY, ASK YOURSELF: "What have I done today that was positive for myself, that helped me grow?" Acknowledge what you have done, then imagine doing even more wonderful things for yourself tomorrow.

Flexibility of Response

Our response to an event is more important than the event itself. —Angeles Arrien

Perhaps for the first thirty or forty years of life, a particular way of doing things brought us the desired result. For instance, striving harder led to good grades in school and promotions at work. Then, at some point, it stopped working; illness or injury occurred. At that point, striving will not solve the problem. Only a change in how we approach life can offer the possibility of healing.

As a biofeedback therapist, using instruments to monitor muscle tension, I observed again and again how inflexibility is an invitation for illness or injury. We have 500 muscles; overusing fifty of them while underusing the other 450 may cause injury. "Repetitive strain injury" is caused by making the same movements, most commonly with the wrists and hands while working at a computer keyboard, over and over again, seven hours a day, five days a week. Usually this repetitive muscular pattern is accompanied by a less conscious, though equally ingrained pattern of tightening the shoulders under the daily pressure of work. This "stereotypic response pattern" must be varied, or broken, in order for healing to occur.

Yoga teaches symmetry: Most positions will be balanced by their mirror image. Yet when working, for many tasks we use just our dominant arm and hand. An exercise program that strengthens the whole body may be an important part of healing. Becoming aware of, and releasing, unconscious muscle tensions may also help. Sometimes a career change is necessary.

Since the body and the mind are so closely interwoven, habitual limited movement patterns lead to limitation in our thinking patterns. Don't be guilty of failure of the imagination! Give yourself permission to break some self-imposed rules.

A person who eats the same foods (such as wheat and dairy products) every day with little variation will not only fail to receive all the needed nutrients but may become hypersensitive or allergic to the overused foods. Improved health results when greater variety is added to the diet.

Boredom is toxic.

Boredom results from being closed to the voices, sights, metaphors, and teachings that are present in the world around us all the time. There is always something to learn if we open our senses and empty our minds. If we have only a limited repertoire of responses to challenging situations, we will be more reactive than responsive. An old behavior, perhaps learned in childhood and repeated many times, is used automatically, without a sense of choice. The "fight or flight response" is innate in all mammals confronted with a threat (whether real or only perceived). In humans, "flight" may mean avoidance and denial of situations or feelings; "fight" may mean only angry words rather than physical aggression. Unfortunately, many of us fall into one of these modes when we perceive a threat. These limited responses undermine close, intimate, loving, nourishing connections and lead to problems in interpersonal relationships.

Alternatives include communication of feelings, wishes, or needs, and negotiation of win-win solutions. Another possibility is to shift perception so that a threat is viewed as an opportunity or a challenge. Once when I was fuming over having been issued a parking ticket, I decided to pretend it was my voluntary, magnanimous donation to the city for its parks and recreation services. Instantly, I felt better!

How flexible is your language? Certain words, such as "never," "always," and "can't," as well as dichotomies like "right/wrong" and "good/bad," lock us into rigid thought patterns. The more options we have, the greater our flexibility. Having two choices gives me a little flexibility, but having three choices gives me a lot more. When in a difficult situation, look for three possible responses.

As children, we all felt powerless to some extent in comparison with the adults around us. However, some people tend to

stay stuck in the "helpless" mode throughout adult life. Perhaps they experienced severe trauma as children. For safety or
survival, a child may have been forced to develop a means of
handling the threat: for example, people-pleasing or taking
care of others. The more threat was experienced, the more
strongly ingrained the caretaking behavior becomes, until the
adult comes to believe that disaster will occur if the caretaking
behavior is not done under certain circumstances. Such a
belief clearly prevents flexibility in responding to other people.

Relaxation training can be an important first step for
expanding our options of responding.

Rigid psychological patterns often show up as rigidity and
tension in the muscles. Relaxing the muscles allows more
openness in the mind. We sit, sit, sit all day long. Do some
movements that challenge your body in new ways. Take a yoga,
Feldenkrais, or tai chi class. Walk backwards. Dance! One of
my favorite exercises for flexibility is to move my head as if
tracing a side-lying figure 8 (the infinity symbol) with my nose,
while affirming, "Infinite flexibility." Or try it with your arm
and hand. Then notice the effects on your ways of perceiving
and thinking.

As we leave the fully conscious, alert state and move into
deeper states through relaxation, the censoring and inhibiting
left brain functions are relaxed, allowing for greater play of the
right brain. Spontaneous, usually suppressed images, emotions,
and wisdom can emerge into consciousness. This is why deep
relaxation has been frequently acknowledged as a gateway to
creativity.

By moving into the imaginal realm, all things are possible. If
we can fly in our mind's eye, we can certainly speak up for ourselves, handle difficult people, sing, dance, write books, or heal
injuries. This is sometimes referred to as "mental rehearsal."

Children are particularly adept at making-believe and can be good role models for us adults. Some days I'm better at pretending, other days I'm stuck in adult reality. The next time you find yourself in an argument, try a role reversal. Become your opponent, and argue for his viewpoint, while he takes on your role. This process builds empathy, and can even replace fury with giggles.

Many indigenous cultures understand the wisdom of shifting the frame of reference. For example, the Native American Medicine Wheel tradition involves moving through the circle, or wheel, of the four seasons of each year, each time seeing from a different perspective and with the guidance of different spirit-helpers. The seasons correspond with the four directions, and with our developmental movement through childhood, youth, maturity, and old age. When a person stays in one spot, without movement, no growth can occur. It is against nature, as if the seasons were to stop changing.

The modern Western paradigm, by contrast, has been more linear. We presumed we were making progress by going forward in a straight line. However, this model implies we are always facing in the same direction, which limits our perspective. The symbol of the circular or spiral path, often associated with the feminine, implies a constantly shifting point of view. Thus, we are more likely to stay in a state of empathic relationship to the whole. According to indigenous wisdom, we never travel the circle in the same way twice. The outward-moving line, often associated with the masculine, is susceptible to going far from the center and becoming drastically out of balance. This way of being has led to the environmental disasters we are now facing.

For example, clear-cutting a forest is based on the one-sided view that more profit can be made by taking all the trees from one spot than by selectively cutting a few. But this practice does not look at the situation from the viewpoint of future generations, who will need trees too. Nor does it consider the loss of habitat for other species, the effects on soil stability, or indeed anything but immediate profit. In contrast, most native peoples lived as harmoniously with the natural world as do all other species.

Joanna Macy, author of *Coming Back to Life*, leads groups to practice seeing an issue from four viewpoints: one's own, that of someone diametrically opposed, that of someone living 150 years later, and that of another species.

When faced with an impasse, the inflexible response is to repeat the same behavior, perhaps more forcefully. This is the opposite of creativity. Think of the American trying to speak English to the foreign visitor: When realizing his words have not been understood, the American typically repeats himself, only louder.

What is needed is a shift in perspective, an alternative approach. The good news is that the more we practice this, the more it becomes our natural mode of behavior. As in the old Shaker song, "To turn, turn will be our delight/ Till by turning, turning, we come round right."

HAVE YOU EVER NOTICED your senses shutting down, and with them your creativity? Instead of criticizing yourself, observe with curiosity. Are your muscles uncomfortable and contracted? Have you been sitting in one position too long? Are you cold, hot, thirsty, tired? When was your last full breath? Time for loving kindness to the body! As you open your senses again, how much more can you perceive of the fascinating drama going on around you?

Try doing just one thing a day differently from how you usually do it. Put on the other shoe first. Listen to an unfamiliar radio station. Take a different route home from work. Congratulate yourself for each small shift.

Body Posture

True life is lived when tiny changes occur. —Leo Tolstoy

"Forward head syndrome" is an actual medical condition in which the head is held too far forward, causing pain in the neck and shoulder muscles. If my head is too far forward, I'm leading with my head instead of my heart. I'm going too fast, trying to think my way out of everything, instead of being willing to feel. My body responds by giving me pain messages to let me know that is not the way to live. If I let my head be too far forward, my chest tends to collapse. This closes my heart and simultaneously broadcasts a posture of guardedness, fear, and defeat to the world and to my inner self. Energy needs to travel freely along the spine, and I block it when I hunch forward. If I listen well to my pain messages, I will bring my head back into proper alignment and let my chest come up and open. What can help me to shift this pattern?

• I need to slow down. Easier said than done, in a society that always seems to demand that we do more and more. The key is to be present in the moment. That is the only way to have enough time. Taking a conscious breath is the best way I know to become present in the moment. Nature, which obeys no clocks, can entrain me into its naturally slower rhythm. Thich Nhat Hanh, a Vietnamese Zen Buddhist teacher, advises us to let the phone ring a couple of times while taking a slow breath, letting it be a "mindfulness bell," a reminder to become present, before answering. How I breathe is always within my power to choose. Fast breathing creates more hurry and stress, while slow breathing facilitates a shift into relaxation and calm.

- I can begin acting as if I believe in myself. How would a woman stand if she believed she had something worthwhile to offer?
- I can cultivate courage. If it feels scary and vulnerable to have an open chest and to let my heart lead me, what are my fears? Is there a way to perceive the world as a friendlier place? Maya Angelou says that acting with courage "puts starch in your spine."
- As I walk, I repeat a mantra: "Long neck, heavy shoulders, lifted chest, relaxed spine."
- I can let gravity do the work. To help open up and relax contracted muscles, I can lie on the floor with a rolled-up blanket or towel vertically along my spine.
- I can enlist a friend to take sneaky pictures of me at home, at work, playing, walking. The sneakier, the better. A video-camera might be even more revealing. Unconscious postures have the most power; that power diminishes when I learn what they are.
- I can love myself and radiate that love outward.

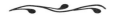

TRY THIS EXERCISE: Slouch into a depressed body posture and try to think positive thoughts, such as "I have gifts to offer the world." Now stand in a confident, upright posture and notice whether it becomes easier to think positively.

Warming

Just explore, without judging your performance.

—Erik Peper

How do I open my heart to myself? Everyone tells us to love ourselves. One of the most basic ways to do that is to start with loving these bodies we live in. When I feel cold, I breathe shallowly; my whole body contracts as my muscles tense against the chill. Allowing my body to be warm and to relax is a simple and very basic way of loving it.

Biofeedback training includes the use of temperature sensors to monitor and display second-by-second changes in skin temperature. When I first began to work with biofeedback, I learned that it is possible to warm up the tips of my fingers by imagining the blood flowing there. For me, it works best to let my shoulder muscles relax completely, breathe slowly and deeply, and become quiet and calm. Then, I imagine my heart sending out loving energy, warmth, and nurturance to my whole body.

Warm hands are receiving the natural healing power of our blood flow. Cool hands may be a signal that the nervous system is stressed. Simply practicing conscious breathing will probably result in warmer hands. Raising our hand temperature at will lets us experience the ability we all have to influence our physical state with mental intention.

To have warm hands, do the practical things first. Make sure your whole body is warm enough. You can warm your hands best when your entire body is at a comfortable temperature; this may mean that you need to dress more warmly than other people. Dressing in layers that you can peel off and add back on helps to maintain the temperature that is comfortable for you. Part of being kind to yourself is attending to your unique needs. A warm hat and scarf can prevent heat loss when you are outdoors. Wearing gloves outside can help, too. Fingerless gloves make it easier to continue using your fingers. When I'm outside and feel cold, it often helps to get moving and exercise to warm myself up. Your hands help you every day in so many ways. Take care that those dear hands don't get chilled. Check in with them often; be kind to them.

Here's a way to bring awareness right into the tips of your fingers: Tap your fingertips together fifty times or so, then rest your hands in your lap, paying attention to the sensations in your fingertips all the while. You may be aware of tingling sensations caused by blood circulating into your fingers.

To help you warm your hands, believe in your own ability to self-direct, to self-regulate.

Feel the warmth at the center of your chest and breathe with it.

Send warm feelings from your heart to your hands.

Trust yourself.

Be willing to let go.

Hands will warm.

Can you recall a place where you felt radiant warmth and happiness to your core? Is it a vast white beach, with green mountains looming in the distance and the ocean shimmering with light? Or perhaps a mountain meadow with birds singing pure notes through clear air, while the sun pours its light into the sweet-smelling pine trees? Such memories can evoke all the healing power of the actual place.

Move your focus from your head (thoughts) to your heart (feelings). Breathe and imagine a furnace glowing in your chest, hot red coals warming and brightening with each slow deep breath, like oxygen being added to a fire; exhale this glowing warmth down your arms. Imagine someone or something you love unconditionally: It could be your grandmother, a purring cat, a small smiling child. Breathe with it; join it; love it. Wrap your loved one in the warm feeling. Include yourself in the warmth. All transformative change flows through the heart.

Releasing the Past

The past is over, it can touch me not.

—A *Course in Miracles*

Our body organs and cells hold memories of emotions not fully experienced, due to fear of being overwhelmed, conditioning not to feel, and not being allowed to be angry or sad. Our bodies function as a storage vault for these emotions, keeping them safe until we feel strong enough to experience them fully.

When we are able to resolve these feelings or see events with a different perspective, we can heal our past. It recently dawned on me that whatever is going on in my back has to do with what is behind me, my past. Pain in my back then becomes a reminder of what needs to be felt more fully and released. It took three whiplash experiences to keep bringing my attention back to my thoracic spine, where an old emotional injury was being stored.

Wayne Dyer says that our past experience is like the wake of a boat. The boat is powered forward by the energy and intention of the present moment, not by the wake, which is only a trail. The past thus has no power to shape our present experience except through our beliefs about it.

The nature of our bodies' wounds is to heal, unless we keep

reopening them. To the extent that we learn to use the power of the present moment, the past becomes less important. The usefulness of the past is in giving us insight that prepares us for taking our next steps.

What story do you tell yourself and others about any past experience? I started thinking about the "story" after a trip to Hawaii, when I was showing my friends the photographs I had taken. I noticed that what I told people about my vacation was strongly influenced by the photographs I'd taken, and I didn't even mention places where I hadn't taken pictures. After a visit to an intentional community in Oregon, I realized that I could make my friends believe I'd had either a terrible time or a wonderful time, depending on what aspects of the place I chose to mention. If I describe a relationship by saying "It was a failure," I'll have a harder time letting go than if I say, "I've learned and grown, and moved on." We are the editors of our own life stories.

As an experiment, try casting yourself as the wily, creative hero who brings life and fun, rather than the hapless victim or the tragic self-sacrificing martyr.

Surgery

There is a culture where, when a person has certain problems with his heart, an amazing ceremony is performed. The ill person is stripped of his clothes and isolated from his family. Dressed in strange greenish costumes that cover even their faces and feet, medicine men use powerful gases to place the sufferer into a deathlike state so that he cannot even breathe without help. Then, they cut into his chest and make his heart stop beating while they extract pieces or insert foreign objects into it.

Yes, this is our culture, and thousands of open-heart surgeries are performed each year. There are often alternatives to surgery (for example, Dr. Dean Ornish's "Opening the Heart" program for bypassing surgery); sometimes, however, surgery is the best or the only choice. The good news is that people can take an active role in preparing themselves for surgery, resulting in less anxiety, decreased pain, more rapid recovery, and shorter hospital stays.

In the current medical system, patients give all power to the surgeon and are passive. Feeling helpless is hard on our nervous systems and immune systems; when we are anxious, our ability to heal is diminished. Research in psychoneuroimmunology has revealed links between anxiety, helplessness, and suppression of the immune response. A study by Janice Kiecolt-Glaser on medical students revealed that their immune responses were lower right before exams than at the start of the semester. However, immune activity was boosted by a mere twenty minutes of guided deep relaxation. Other studies indicate that a feeling of powerlessness, a "hopeless-helpless" attitude, leads to a decrease in immune functioning.

At New York Presbyterian Hospital, thanks to its Complementary Medicine services, patients have access to classes on hypnosis, breath, guided imagery, and meditation. Jery Whitworth, R.N., executive director of the department, states that patients who use these services report that their stress drops (by an average of 69 percent); reported pain decreases by 57 percent. "People who have done mind/ body preparation for surgery usually need less anesthesia during the operation and less pain medicine afterwards," says Steven Gurgevich, Ph.D., a psychologist who teaches self-hypnosis and provides audio-tapes to patients at Dr. Andrew Weil's Integrative Medicine Clinic in Tucson, Arizona. These patients also have fewer complications and recover faster.

The first step in regaining your personal power is to lower your anxiety, through a daily practice of relaxation and healing imagery. There are many relaxation tapes available, some of which are specifically designed to enhance surgical outcomes; I would recommend tapes by Belleruth Naparstek or Peggy Huddleston. Visualizing favorable outcomes, perhaps with the help of a tape, overcomes fear and programs our bodies to respond in desirable ways. Peggy Huddleston suggests imagining yourself saying, "Everything went well, I feel fine," right after the operation. Next, imagine the healing process taking place in your body; and finally, see and feel yourself doing something you love, fully enjoying life. As with any imagery process, the power lies in regular practice (twice a day for a week or two before surgery, if possible), and vivid, multisensory detail, so that it engages you emotionally.

Creating a circle of support, Huddleston's third step, is very valuable. Ask your family and friends to wrap you in a warm blanket of love and good wishes, half an hour before the time your surgery is scheduled. It gives them something more constructive to do than worry about you, and many studies now demonstrate the powerful healing effects of prayer or loving thoughts from a distance. (See *Healing Words* by Dr. Larry Dossey.) You can also arrange for a loved one to be with you just before and after the operation.

Bringing your vague worries into full conscious awareness so that you can examine them realistically and perhaps talk them over with a counselor, or in a support group, is healing in itself. Taking a deeper look at the part of your body which is ill, as discussed in previous chapters, and even having a dialogue with your symptom, may reveal emotional issues which you can begin to express and address. When anxiety arises, breathe slowly and trade in your worry thought for an image of yourself fully healed.

Prior to surgery and also while under anesthesia, our minds are as suggestible as if we were in a hypnotic state. In a study by Dr. Henry Bennett, a group of patients were told, fifteen minutes before surgery, that they could direct their bloodflow away from the site of the surgical incision. This group lost on average only 500 cc of blood, while a control group averaged a 900 cc blood loss. Dr. McLintock and others at the Royal Infirmary in Glasgow, Scotland, studied women undergoing abdominal hysterectomy. Those who listened to a tape of "positive therapeutic suggestions" while under anesthesia required 24 percent less pain medication the day after surgery than patients who listened to a blank tape.

You can create a tape for yourself with suggestions on it such as: "I have control over my blood flow. My blood moves away from the incision site, and returns after the stitches are in place." "After my operation I'll be hungry, my stomach will gurgle, and I will urinate easily." "My body is healing rapidly and well. I feel comfortable." It is becoming commonplace for patients to bring battery-powered cassette players and headphones into operating rooms.

The wife of an 81-year-old man called me after he had a kidney removed. They had attended Peggy Huddleston's "Prepare for Surgery, Heal Faster" workshop, which I am certified to teach. "I just want to let you know that it really worked! My husband breezed through that surgery, in spite of his heart and lung problems. Afterwards, the nurses and doctors couldn't believe how little pain medication he was using, less than four milligrams of morphine and a little tylenol. They kept asking, 'Don't you want more pain medication?' And the healing! He was supposed to be in the hospital for seven days, and he was out in four. They told him he'd be in rehab for a week, but it was less than four days."

She went on to describe how her husband had listened to the relaxation tape and visualized the healing outcomes he wished for. The night before surgery, he "said goodbye" to his kidney and thanked it for everything it had done for him. He also gave a "pep talk" to his other kidney, telling it to get ready to do the work of two. The couple asked their friends, family, and members of their church group to send "a warm red blanket of love with a valentine heart on it," since his surgery was scheduled for February 15.

Although she encountered initial resistance from the medical staff, she was able to persuade the anesthesiologist to use healing statements during the operation. The anesthesiologist even added a suggestion: "You no longer smoke cigarettes." During the operation, the patient listened to a special tape his wife had made for him which said, "As the kidney leaves you, so does your desire to smoke." A week after the surgery, he had not even asked for a cigarette.

Surgery need not create feelings of helplessness and anxiety when you play an active role in your preparation and healing process.

For an easy step-by-step guide to mind-body techniques for surgery, I highly recommend Peggy Huddleston's book and audiotape entitled *Prepare for Surgery, Heal Faster.*

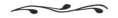

Illness as a Rite of Passage

When a ritual is used to mark an important transition from one condition to another, it may be called a "rite of passage." An example is the transition from childhood to adulthood, marked in some traditional societies with a Vision Quest. There are three phases:

• separation (taking leave of one's previous way of life)
• transition (introspective, alone time, perhaps in an altered state of consciousness induced by fasting)
• return (re-entry into a new life).

Transitions always involve both losses and gains. Hence, the rite of passage is a symbolic death and re-birth. The youth entering adulthood takes leave of the child self and, after a period of solitary fasting and visioning, is welcomed back to his or her community, celebrated as an adult with a sense of mission resulting from the vision received. He or she may take on a new name representing the wisdom gained.

As Achterberg, Dossey, and Kokmeier point out in *Rituals of Healing*, serious illness, injury, or surgery may also be viewed as rites of passage. Sometimes a breakdown is necessary so that a new order can take shape in our body-mind. Inside the cocoon, the form of the caterpillar is completely obliterated. What if, instead of trying to return to a life exactly the same as it was before, we treated these events as a transition into a different way of being? We might prepare ourselves for rebirth into a new, spiritually deeper experience of life.

Although illness or surgery includes losses, there are also gains. The transition phase is a period of "cocoon" time, where the person is relieved of life's usual responsibilities in order to recuperate. Many people have stated that this time provided a precious opportunity to slow down and reflect upon life's purpose and meaning. There are also times—for example, after a mastectomy—when the loss seems much more tangible than the gain. A ritual can make a difference. A woman who belonged to a support group was treated to a ceremonial welcome after her mastectomy, honored for her courage, and given a new status within the group.

A Circle of Strengths

Group ceremonies can reduce the anxiety of a person who is ill, thus enabling better healing. In her wonderful book, *Kitchen Table Wisdom*, Rachel Naomi Remen describes a ritual whereby a group can provide a tangible expression of their support to a person who is about to have surgery. A special stone is passed around, and while holding the stone, each person speaks about a time of calling upon a resource or an inner strength to survive a crisis. The stone, imbued with all the strength of the circle, is then kept by the person and may even be brought into surgery. This physical embodiment of the group's energy "makes caring visible."

When a member of our Community Circle was about to have surgery, the group offered many stories of our sources of strength while the stone was passed around. We shared anecdotes about prayer, staying centered, letting go, single-mindedness, beauty, nature, mystery, humor, surrender, and admitting the fear.

When facing a similar surgery, D. S. was helped by his son's prayers for him in a sweat lodge, and a prayer bundle made especially for him by his son.

Confronted by a burning car on one side and a charging buffalo on the other, F. K. realized that the only way to go was forward, and went for it singlemindedly!

While walking on a windy trail with a dangerous knife-edge pass, K. L. was able to focus and center himself to stay safe.

When going in for laser surgery on her eyes, I. H. was able to let go of needing to know in advance what to expect. As a result, she was free of worry.

In the midst of a relationship crisis, M. K. put on earphones and listened to a favorite section of the Bach St. Matthew Passion, twenty times. The music helped her transcend her problems and tap into the magic of the larger reality.

Following an angry outburst at my sister during a summer solstice camping trip in Yosemite, I felt completely cleansed by a drenching hike past Vernal Falls, and our relationship began to heal.

During the difficulties of the Great Peace March of 1986, T. A. learned to accept the larger pattern, to trust the mystery that transcends all ordinary standards.

Immediately after a very traumatic car accident, E. L. recalls that she was able to say to another friend who was less injured, "How's that for one-upmanship?" She experienced the painful recovery as an intense growth period, and felt very peaceful, realizing that she would be fine even if she were to die.

D. B. got over her shame about her fear of flying, and stopped forcing herself to fly; she took trains instead. As she got to know her fear, she became curious about it. When she finally decided to try flying again, she was able to admit her anxiety to a stewardess and received support.

After taking part in this ritual, we all felt whole. We felt bonded with each other on a deeper level, and we experienced the joy of being able to offer something valuable to our friend.

Emotions and Pain

Anger

*Deep feelings are the voices that need to be heard and
expressed to find our transformation. The only feelings
that don't change are the ones we don't let go of.*

—Anne Brener

Anger and frustration can do a lot of mischief in our
bodies as well as in our relationships. Living fully
includes getting in closer touch with feelings. For
some of us, emotions flow spontaneously, while for others, it
may take patient invitation to access what we feel. Most of us
were not permitted to express our anger, when we were growing up. As adults we tend to judge ourselves for feeling angry,
and/or pretend we're not really angry. If I shut down and reject
my anger, I force the energy inside myself, where it creates tension and pressure. I then feel tired and depleted, and an illness
may result. An alternative is to breathe, let myself feel the
anger, and ask, "What constructive thing can I do with this
intense energy?" I might use it to mow the lawn, pull weeds (an
excellent metaphor for me), or clean house. The energy of
anger is like fire, which, although it can wreak destruction if
ignored or handled carelessly, can be used constructively for
warming a house or cooking.

Sometimes, I breathe deeply and move around, stomping or

punching the air, until I feel a release. Our emotions are like waves of energy. When we can experience them fully, we can move right through them. Breath is also like a wave; by breathing with our emotions, instead of suppressing them and holding our breath, we can move through them in a natural way. At first I was afraid to be that present with my emotions. I imagined that they would become so overwhelming I wouldn't be able to bear it. I have often been surprised at how quickly the feelings peak in intensity and then disperse when I'm willing to breathe and move them through.

Taking a little space for myself when I am angry helps me immensely. If I'm not ready to communicate rationally, I can take a walk and breathe until I feel calmer. A new perspective will often dawn on me during those few minutes of reprieve from the situation. While walking, I'm not trying to "stuff" the anger down out of sight, or distract myself from it. I'm being with it, rather than acting on it.

Once I had a houseguest who became quite ill and needed a lot of help from me. I felt imposed upon and angry, yet I knew it was not his fault. To handle my feelings, I excused myself for a quick bike ride. While I was pedaling like a demon, I growled and cursed aloud. When I returned home, I was much more calm, patient, and understanding. A friend told me about a woman who puts her sons to work chopping wood, instead of punishing them, when they have violated an agreement. This struck me as a great way to let the boys work off their anger, while also contributing useful work as a form of restitution.

Having an angry outburst can feel very cleansing and may offer a sense of relief. Unfortunately, exploding my anger at other people can also keep me stuck in it. The other person typically reacts with defensiveness or returns the anger, and conflict escalates instead of being resolved. Also, I continue to practice and reinforce the habit of hostile behavior and blaming others. In anger, I close my heart, thinking I'm punishing the other person; but in reality it punishes me more. What joy can I feel when my heart is closed?

Thich Nhat Hanh suggests that we hold our anger, or other uncomfortable emotions, as we might cradle a crying baby in our arms, being fully present. A baby begins to feel better just by being held in a loving way. As the mother attends to the baby, she will soon discover the cause of the crying, whether it was hunger or a wet diaper. Similarly, as we attend deeply to our feelings, we discover their true source.

Anger is one of the disguises my fear hides behind. When I look more deeply at the anger, I often see a frightened little person behind the tough angry mask. Admitting my fear to myself dissolves a lot of the anger. Speaking about the fear to the other person involved is harder than blaming and accusing him, but usually gets much better results.

For example, I used to get furious with my husband if we were having guests over and he didn't help me prepare. I was afraid that I would be overwhelmed with too much to do, it wouldn't get done, and our friends would not have a good time. When I finally learned to express the fears, instead of calling him lazy and selfish, it became easier for him to assist me. He was able to explain that he had avoided helping me because I acted so stressed and pressured and tended to boss him around.

Often part of the problem is my tendency to hold on to anger, self-righteously proclaiming: "I'm entitled to my anger!" But anger is like a hot potato: If I hold it tightly, it burns me. One technique I use is to exhale and pretend I'm pushing away the person who's bugging me, or the traffic, or whatever the problem is. I feel the anger energy inside me, visualize it, summon it all up into my lungs, and exhale it out, picturing it leaving me.

My current favorite image is that of composting my anger putting it with the kitchen scraps and grass clippings so it can later help grow vegetables.

Don't judge yourself for feeling angry. It's a signal that something needs adjustment. It is helpful to notice whenever someone crosses a boundary you have. Anger is often a response to feeling trespassed against. Sometimes the anger is at yourself, for not honoring those boundaries enough to make them clear to others. It's your right and responsibility to draw a line, to respect your own needs, wishes, and even preferences. The more you respect them, the more others will too. By having invisible or uncertain boundaries, we invite others to cross them. Let go of any guilt about having boundaries. We all need them. Sometimes saying no to another person is the nicest thing I can do for him (although neither of us may realize it at the time).

When a boundary has been crossed, it is useful to practice assertive communication and empathic listening skills: State your feelings without blaming or judging the other person. It's much easier to hear "I feel hurt and angry that you didn't call," than "You should have called me." By stating feelings, there is no dispute about right or wrong. Feelings simply *are*; they are your truth. Also, stating feelings places you in the "vulnerable" position, so the other person doesn't need to feel defensive.

Another person or his actions or a situation is not what "makes" us angry. It is actually our own thought, beliefs, evaluations and judgments that create the anger. "It's unfair" is an evaluation that creates anger. Many spiritual teachings, such as *A Course in Miracles*, encourage us to see others' actions as being the best they could do at that moment, as an expression of their pain, even a cry for help and understanding. Instead of responding to someone's attacking words with an angry retort, try an empathic acknowledgment of his or her feelings: "Are you angry because you're needing more cooperation from your co-workers?"

Sometimes my anger is triggered when someone's behavior reminds me of a part of myself I don't approve of very much. If I can forgive or accept that aspect of myself, the anger dissipates. On a backpacking trip with a woman friend, I was feeling annoyed with her frequently. At every point where a decision needed to be made, whether it was which fork in the trail to take, or how long to boil the noodles, she seemed to insist on being "right." Just as I was about to point out to her that she had a problem, my self-righteousness was punctured by a small voice inside that asked me, "Why does it matter to you whether she gets to be right?" Inwardly, I protested, "But don't I get to be right, just once in awhile?" Then it dawned on me: What I found so irritating in my friend's behavior was exactly the issue I needed to work on in myself. My anger evaporated.

The more I catch on to my ego games, the more I can laugh at them. Nothing defuses anger like laughter.

A wise four-year-old taught me about playing dinosaurs. We could pretend to fight and be violent, but it was just play. Dinosaurs are extinct, so they are a good choice (since we'll be extinct too if we don't learn to manage our anger without violence). At the same time, there is value in occasional ferocity. Ferocity can be an aspect of leadership and strength; it lends us courage and makes us feel strong; and it may even prevent actual violence.

CONSIDER:
- When do you experience anger?
- What need is being unmet, or what boundary crossed?
- How can you take care of your needs?

Freedom from Fear

> *Leap, and the net will appear.*   —Julia Cameron

> *The way toward freedom from a situation often lies in acceptance of the situation.*   —Rachel Naomi Remen

How helpless and frightened I feel on a dark night when my flashlight batteries are dead—or when I hear an ominous rustling outside my tent! We can develop courage by spending time in nature where things are less predictable than they are in our human-made world. On the other hand, being close to the ground can be deeply comforting. Is it possible that much of our fear is caused by our disconnection from the natural world? A sense of belonging is the greatest antidote to fear.

Fear may also come up as we begin to feel more, as well as whenever we begin to make changes and leave familiar habits behind. Remember: Feel the fear, don't feed the fear. It has been said that "Fear is excitement without the breath." So, when fear arises, the first thing to do is to breathe slowly and consciously, while letting the feelings flow through you. A few long, slow exhalations (through the nose or pursed lips) are amazingly effective in managing feelings of panic. In the biofeedback clinic, I have watched how people can lower their systolic blood pressure by twenty points or more within a minute or two, just by breathing slowly and comfortably. One man remarked, after watching his blood pressure come down to normal, "This way of breathing is like Valium!"

Locate the fear in your body. Where do you constrict, contract, close down? Breathe into those areas, as best you can. Feel the fear, observe it, don't run away from it, and see if it's okay to do what you need to do while feeling afraid. This takes lots of experimentation and practice and creativity. Remember that small steps work best. Each small success leads to increased belief in your ability, increased self-esteem, greater likelihood of another victory.

If you try to move too fast, to "tough it through," and you get hurt or really scared, you will be discouraged from trying again. Learn to relax, exhale, and reassure yourself during and after each baby step. Impatience is our biggest enemy, and it usually comes bolstered by a lot of "shoulds": "You should be able to drive across that bridge," "You shouldn't have to rely on other people to help you," "You should already be over this by now."

Try speaking more kindly and compassionately to yourself. Self-criticism keeps us stuck. Self-acceptance leads to change. The best antidote to panic that I know of is kindness to myself. Buying into others' restrictions, and imposing them on myself, puts me in jail. My fear keeps me trying to be respectable and prevents me from being real.

One of my biggest fears is the fear of looking like a fool. Fear of what others think has stopped me from doing countless worthwhile things, like teaching classes ("What if they find out I'm not an expert on this yet?") The times I've made real progress have been when living my dreams was more important than whether people laughed at me!

Julia Butterfly, the amazing young woman who climbed up a giant redwood tree to prevent clearcutting by Maxxam Corporation in an old-growth forest in northern California, and stayed there for over two years, has a lot to teach us about dealing with fear. During the violent storms of *El Niño* in the winter of 1998, on her platform 180 feet from the ground, she feared for her life. In desperation, she asked the tree for guidance. The tree's response was that she did not have to try to be strong and tough, but instead to be flexible like a tree in a storm. The tree does not resist, but bends with the wind. This attitude is present in Julia's approach to the loggers: She does not place herself in opposition to them, but appeals to our common interest in preserving a viable forest.

Are you living in Scare-city? Fear arises when we perceive a scarcity of time, love, money—whatever we think we need. Fear itself impoverishes us by preventing us from living joyously. There is no lack of what is truly important and valuable. When you feel stuck in scarcity, try giving something away. Native American teacher ChoQosh Au-Ho-Oh tells a beautiful story about a time when she and her daughter had very little money. They got a big lift in spirits by buying two dozen inexpensive roses and placing a rose at each door on their block late at night for the occupant to find the next morning.

When I catch myself being greedy, it's usually because of fear: fear of "not getting enough," or fear of an emotion trying to come through. Stinginess with my time comes from a fearful belief that I don't have enough of it.

"NO FEAR, NO FEAR." Those are the beautiful words my Higher Self murmurs sweetly in my ear at times of need.

Malidoma Somé, a teacher of West African traditional ways, suggests that we ask an ancestor for assistance whenever needed. "There's a high unemployment rate on the other side," he says. "The ancestors love being given a job. But they can't help you if you don't ask." I decided that whenever I felt really frightened, I would inwardly call on my mother, asking her to take my fear from me. It works!

Very few people hurt those who are close to them out of meanness; they do it out of fear. When our mother became critically ill, my brother, sister, and I flew to Boston. We were all terribly afraid of losing her. There were many tasks to be handled, but my sister was so emotionally distraught that I was afraid to give her any responsibility. Very hurt, she protested, "I'm not an invalid." I snapped impatiently, "Just go spend time with Dad." My fears prevented me from being kinder.

Fear leads to the desire to control, to remove others' choices, rather than trusting them. It is the opposite of love. When we act from love, we can give people choices, without attaching our happiness to which choice they make. Loving behavior does not include attempting to manipulate, control, or influence, even for the other's welfare. An exception is with children, where control may be necessary to protect them from harm, for instance, grabbing a child who is running out into the street.

Powerlessness, which leads to violence, results from the belief that there are no choices. Whenever you notice yourself feeling powerless or stuck, look for the second and third possibility. Think of the symbol for change: the triangle. It's no accident that the triangle, with its three points, is considered a sacred shape. When you feel like a victim, ask yourself what your choices are, and look for three of them. "I could choose to do it this way, OR that way, OR the other way." Perceiving more options can be the golden "OR" that helps you row your boat to the other side.

Choices give us freedom. Oh, Freedom! True freedom includes liberation from addictions, which are our self-imposed limitations. Addictions can be a short tether, and sometimes a heavy load. Our addictions are those things that keep us numb enough not to feel our true feelings of pain and joy, and thus keep us from being fully alive and aware. If we're addicted to material comforts, we can't go very far—we can't sleep on the ground if we're addicted to a soft bed. We restrict our possibilities of traveling or of trying anything new if we're hooked on predictability or staying in control. We're limited in our ability to explore career paths if we're attached to having a certain income. Addiction to being right and never making mistakes limits us extremely.

Freedom is also liberation from fears. Many fears are focussed on the possibility that one of our addictive "needs" (demands) will not be met. Yet without risk and trust, how can natural miracles happen to us?

A most miraculous experience occurred several years ago when I truly trusted a vision. One night I was not sleeping well, and in a half-awake, half-dreaming state I became aware of a woman talking to me. Although I caught only a few phrases, I was filled with the exciting conviction that I would soon have a new, wonderful place to live. The words were "glen" and "X-ing." That week, in a playful mood, I began exploring streets with the word "glen" in their names, or with a river glen near-by. One street even had "X-ing" signs for river crossings, but nothing quite fit. Unsure how to proceed, I picked up a classi-fied section, but the feeling in my gut quickly told me that would not be helpful. However, I began packing a few boxes, because the conviction was still there. I even told a few friends that I was expecting to move soon, although I didn't know where yet! One evening at a party, a friend of a friend shook her head and said, "I just don't understand it; my tenant of ten years in my cottage out back wants to move, and she's only given me two weeks' notice." Without having laid eyes on the cottage, I felt that it was to be my new home. A few days later, when I saw it, I gasped with joy. Fresh green unmowed grass was growing all around, pale lavender wisteria was cascading from the roof, and a tall pine tree stood in front. Oh yes, there was a creek that flowed past the house next door. In this effort-less manner my new home came to me.

Examine your fears: fears of others' judgments (and subse-quent abandonment); fears of your own judgments; fears of hurting another's feelings; fears of being hurt. Address these fears by communicating with the other people involved. Ask "Would you be upset/hurt/angry at me if I _____?" "How strongly do you feel about _____?" "I'm feeling confused, can we discuss what's going on?"

Honest communication about feelings may feel scary, but it is our greatest safety. Often I need to start by acknowledging to myself what I'm feeling fearful about. "Name that fear" is the game. Admitting it to myself can be a big relief; admitting it to someone else may be a relief to that other person, as well as to me.

What if there were truly nothing to fear? What if everything that occurred was helping us learn the things we most need and want to know?

Years ago, when I was in college, I was sitting at my desk with my mind wandering away from my book when suddenly I felt as though I had been struck by a bolt of lightning through the top of my head. With this intense cracking open of my consciousness came the unshakeable knowledge that I was *free!* I could dance in the streets! I wept for joy at this sud-den awareness of my true state of complete liberation. Although I did not go dancing in the street, and am often quite cautious, I know deeply now that the only force that restricts me is my own fear. And I know that freedom is not only about dancing with wild abandon, but also about having choices in how to offer my gifts to the world.

Try finishing this sentence: "If I couldn't fail, I would
_____."

Pain and Sensitivity

Pain is a signal that some definition of me, whether physi-
cal or mental, is in conflict with something else.
                                        —Richard Moss, M.D.

Whatever hurts in your body, focus on relaxing it and sending love to it many times a day. Healing comes through
bringing love and awareness to the part that is in pain—not
hating it, disowning it, or distracting yourself from it.

Does your posture support you and feel comfortable?
Whenever you are not using a chronically tense muscle
group—really relax it. Relax deeply at least twenty minutes
each day, perhaps with a tape (see Resources). Also, take
many shorter mini-rests. Notice whenever your painful area
feels good, even if it's only for a few seconds at a time, and
notice what you did or thought or felt to create that.

Every morning, take some slow deep breaths before getting
out of bed. If you wake up with pain, imagine breathing in and
out through the painful area. If you start feeling tense as soon
as you wake up, this slow breathing will help you to undo that
tension habit, which is very much related to chronic pain. As
you are breathing in and out of the tense areas, ask yourself:
"What am I feeling tense or anxious about?" If you are worry-
ing about your performance, reassure yourself by saying, "I
always do my best," or "I accept myself just as I am." Write
down your feelings as a way of honoring and accepting them.
You may discover that you start experiencing them differently.

A wonderful process used by Jon Kabat-Zinn, author of *Full Catastrophe Living*, in his work with chronic pain sufferers, is called "body scanning." Go through your whole body, slowly imagining breathing in and out of each part, including the painful area; treat it just the same as any other region. Observe the sensations, open to them, soften and let go each time you breathe out. Flow into calmness and stillness. Notice your thoughts and emotions, and let go of them without judgment. Expand and become larger than the pain. Notice all the parts of you that are not experiencing pain.

When pain is severe, direct your attention gently and firmly on and into the pain. Don't try to stop or escape it; stop labeling it as "bad." Just observe it, one moment at a time. Find out about it. Notice what you are saying to yourself about it, and realize that the negative judgments or anger may be making the pain worse. Release the thoughts and just breathe with the sensations.

Whenever you make movements that affect your painful area (which may be very frequently), put your mind on your breathing and attempt to keep a slow, smooth flow of air going in and out. In general, try to exhale through the painful or effortful movements.

If you have a stiff or sore neck or suffer from tension headaches, turn your head from side to side, with your eyes open, at least twice an hour, or any time you feel stressed or upset. As you do, say inwardly: "I can see other viewpoints," or "I can see this situation differently." If your head feels congested, distribute some mental energy and heat to your hands, by getting up from your desk and doing some physical work. Or, you could close your eyes and imagine heat and energy pouring down from your head, through your shoulders and arms, and into your hands.

We have all abused our bodies through unconscious habitual patterns such as tensing. Dwelling on guilt feelings about these patterns does not help. Just apologize to your body, begin to notice when the harmful patterns show up, and choose differently. As we become aware of our habits, we have immense power to change.

Honor your body's subtle messages. Don't be tough on your body, and it won't be tough on you. Be gentle. Celebrate and value your ability to pick up small signals from your body that all is not well, so your body won't have to turn up the volume. Many people with migraine headache learn to recognize the typical pattern of stress that portends the onset of a headache, and even become aware of subtle sensations which are unusual. By taking time out and resting, they can diminish the severity or even prevent the migraine completely.

When I was a child, my mother used to tease me about not being tough enough: "You delicate little flower," she would say, with a hint of sarcasm. I've gradually learned to protect my thin skin not by "armoring" my body, but rather by putting space around others' judgments or criticisms of me. One way I can do this is to remember that their opinions are not universally shared. Sometimes the person who judges or criticizes me may simply be having a bad day. I learned from Serge King, author of *Urban Shaman*, to neutralize a critical remark by silently praising or appreciating myself.

Remember the story of "The Princess and the Pea"? It reminds us that exquisite sensitivity and subtlety of perception are to be valued. Being ill or in pain may cause heightened awareness, and often illness allows us to take a break from the distractions of daily life, going deeper within. As our sensitivity increases, we become more aware of other subtle occurrences around us, and more open to the many forms of guidance or gentle nudges that the universe is always offering. When we learn to honor and work with our sensitivity, we may be able to detect fluctuations in our energy field and brush them off or ground them out before physical illness develops. Heightened sensitivity can be a means of achieving greater health and well-being.

Slight pain gives us an opportunity to listen to the body's messages in a relatively nonthreatening way. Instead of thinking, "My body is too sensitive; I should be comfortable sitting here," I can view my discomfort as a nudge from my body to do something different. I might shift the focus of my attention, breathe more deeply, or move around more. If I am cold in the shade, I can move to the sun or begin walking briskly to warm myself up. I can appreciate my responsive body for its aliveness and its messages to me. It knows more than I do about my needs as a total being; the key is to trust and act upon that wisdom rather than forcing my body to do what "I" want it to.

The body's discomfort can be a guide to intuition. What movement does your body feel like making? Make that movement and notice your feelings. Where does it lead? Pain is also a gift that protects us from more serious injury, as when we get a slight burn and the pain causes us to draw back from a hot stove. Pain often has a message if we are open to hearing it.

If you need your body's cooperation to get through a challenge, don't shut down your sensitivities. Speak respectfully to your body and ask it to do what you want it to. If you get a clear "no" from your body, don't force it. You may feel tempted to give up because you can't do the things you want and need to do. At those times, take the smallest, slowest steps; be gentle with yourself *and* keep moving, making gradual progress.

Is pain "good for you"? In my opinion, pain is overrated. Suffering is not inherently valuable. What has value is finding the way to transform suffering, discovering the blessing and the learning and the healing. Staying stuck in suffering is not the purpose. Pain offers us an opportunity to learn; it does not force us to learn. Some folks don't learn from pain but simply die with it. In fact—if you feel forced, you probably haven't learned the whole lesson. Part of the lesson might be that we don't need the pain if we're willing to learn in other ways. Change may be frightening, but staying stuck is true suffering. What pain does is to prevent us from sleeping through our lives. It can be a great Awakener. Those who discover these blessings can shine as a light to others, assisting them to overcome similar challenges.

To quote Dr. Christiane Northrup: "The work we do to let go of our suffering diminishes the suffering of the whole universe. When we have room for our own pain, we have room for the pain of others and we actually help 'carry' the suffering of others. Only then can it be transformed into joy."

The Tibetan Buddhists have a practice called *tonglen* that makes use of the pain we all experience, rather than regarding it as useless suffering. Like many other Buddhist practices, it involves the breath. Breathing in, we take on our own suffering, such as a toothache, without judgment, with compassion. Breathing out, we release our acceptance and serenity to the world. Then we progress to breathing in and taking on the similar suffering of others, such as all other people suffering with toothache at this moment. Exhaling, we offer compassion to all those. Finally, we can breathe in the suffering of all beings from any causes, and breathe out our acceptance and compassion to all.

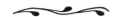

CONSIDER:

- What do you use to dull or diminish your sensitivity? Has it become an addiction?
- Ask your body: "What are you trying to tell me? What do you need me to do differently?" Take the time to listen and observe. Once you get the message, ask yourself whether you are willing to make the necessary changes in your life. Treating your body lovingly, instead of ignoring its grumblings, is a great way to start loving and accepting *all* of yourself.

The Inner Selves

We are complex beings. Within each of us there are many, many aspects, some of which seem to be at war with others. The Inner Guide has been discussed earlier; some may think of this as the "Higher Self." In this section we will explore some of the other characters who inhabit our inner world.

The Inner Critic

> *Compassion for yourself translates into compassion for others.* —Suki Jay Munsell

We all have an Inner Critic: that voice that nags at us, puts us down, tells us we're not good enough. When we were little, our parents or teachers were critical of us, and we developed the habit of criticizing ourselves. When I hear a voice in my head saying "You failed," that's a giveaway that my Critic is speaking. Only the Critic would say that.

Be aware of the Critic's distinctive voice or pattern. Often the Critic masquerades as Reality or Truth and keeps its true identity well hidden. At such times, go cautiously and ask yourself: "Is it possible that there is another way to see this situation?" The tricky part is to remember to ask this question. Ask it whenever you start feeling bad, especially if you are putting yourself down or judging a situation as hopeless.

Know that you can always choose whether or not to tune in on the Critic channel, or some other channel of your mind; don't hesitate to switch channels as soon as you realize you're hearing the Critic. Haven't you spent enough of your life listening to that voice? Perhaps it was useful at one time, and then you may not have realized that you had any other option, but now you know there is a choice. Be aware that you can decide whether or not to listen to the Critic, to believe it, or to act on what it says. Whenever you do make another choice, observe carefully what happens. Although the Critic has always warned you that disaster would ensue if you stopped obeying it, discover whether or not this is true in your experience.

When I listen to my Critic too much, everyone around me starts sounding bossy and critical. I start seeing Critics all around me because I project them from my own mind. Hearing the Critic's judgmental words, I begin using this language toward others, and they in turn feel criticized by me. At such times, try telling your Critic to put earphones on and listen to its favorite music.

When others are angry at me, my Inner Critic arises and says, "See—you did it wrong, you failed to please them." Now, when I hear that, I'm learning to say, "I did the best I could at the time. If they are angry, perhaps it's their problem."

Despite all the abuse my Critic seems to heap upon me, it has a valuable role to play in my life. When I was growing up, its cautions helped me to survive; I need to honor it for that. When the Critic's voice is getting in my way, I sometimes say: "Thank you for your concerns. Please save them for later. I'll check in with you after a while." This frees me from my Critic while I focus on an important situation. Later, I can dialogue with my Critic and ask about its fears. Usually I learn that my

Critic was afraid of a possible negative consequence of my behavior, and was trying to protect me. It's good to define for your Critic what you want its job to be, while setting limits on when you will listen to it.

Once while I was attending a workshop with Barbara Brennan, I was practicing the skill of tuning into other people's energy fields. My Critic was declaring loudly, "You'll never learn how to do that; you have no skill whatsoever!" I thanked it and asked it to be silent for awhile, promising that I would check in later. Much to my surprise, I was then able to do rather accurate readings of two participants in the workshop. On the train ride home, I remembered to check in with my Critic. It brought up a fear of which I had not been consciously aware: that if I were to develop psychic skills, some people would perceive me as weird or crazy, and I might lose certain friends. This was the first time I had ever truly listened to my Critic on my own terms, instead of raging against it or meekly complying with it. I was impressed by its genuine concern for my well-being.

When my Critic is ranting about some error or act of poor judgment I've made, it sometimes works well to outline what I would do differently next time. For instance, when my Critic was berating me over missing the Creek Cleanup Day, I said: "Next time, I will write it down in my schedule. That way I won't miss it or schedule other things for that day."

Sometimes it seems more like a Complainer than a Critic. It's a fearful voice that worries, "You've made the wrong decision, this experience isn't what it should be, you're missing out." The false perception that leads to complaining and criticism is based on the belief that I have to rely only on my own wits and choices (with no help available from Spirit). This calls for a compassionate but firm reply, such as: "Dear Complainer, I'm sorry that this experience isn't quite up to your expectations. But life isn't really about finding the most perfect experiences, it's about making the best of whatever is given. Let's focus on what is delightful instead of what isn't." Fear of missing out can actually cause us to miss out on the present moment! We can never know enough to make the wisest choice at all times, but we can choose to look for the gift.

ASK YOURSELF: What is my Inner Critic trying to protect me from?

The Impartial Witness

> *The witness position is your center—it is like the eye of*
> *the storm.*   —Joan Borysenko

The best balance to the Inner Critic is the Impartial Witness. The role of the Witness is not to judge, compare, criticize, or give orders, but simply to observe with impartiality, detachment, curiosity, even wonder. The Witness might say things like, "Let's take another look" and "Is this the real truth or not?"

Ram Dass tells a story of a farmer with a son and a horse, both of whom give him great joy. One day, the horse runs away, and all the villagers shake their heads in consternation. The farmer says, "We'll see." The next day, his son goes out to search for the horse, and instead comes back with two wild horses, both very splendid. The neighbors say, "What good fortune." The farmer says simply, "We'll see." A few days later, as the son tries to ride one of the wild horses he is thrown off and breaks his leg. "Poor fellow," intone the neighbors, sympathetically. The farmer: "We'll see." The next week, war breaks out and all the young men of draft age are signed up to defend their village; all, that is, except the farmer's son, who is too disabled to fight. "Lucky man!" sigh the villagers. And so on it goes. The farmer, like the Impartial Witness, does not get caught in the emotional roller coaster caused by evaluating each event as good or bad, lucky or unlucky. He observes and accepts what is, without judgment. Therein lies his serenity.

To me, the Witness is like the sky above, observing everything; or like the ancestors looking upon us with unconditional positive regard, and perhaps a touch of fond amusement. Great old trees have this quality of pure awareness, perhaps because they have witnessed so many generations of humans and animals and their dramas. The trees remain unmoved, a stable awareness in times of crisis and storms.

How can we cultivate the Impartial Witness? Thich Nhat Hanh reminds us of the witness quality of quiet water, which we can learn to emulate by quieting our minds, with this meditative phrase: "Breathing in, I see myself as still water. Breathing out, I am reflecting things as they are."

Angeles Arrien advises that our Witness needs to be stronger than our Critic; "Stop feeding your Critic gourmet meals," she says. She suggests that we look at our experiences without exaggeration or diminishment. When I observe myself doing something that appears to have a negative consequence, I am now learning to say, "How interesting! What can I learn here?" The Witness looks with curiosity and a desire to understand; it doesn't attempt to evaluate.

One of the great tasks that I believe we all come here to accomplish is to learn who we are. That sounds funny in a way. Aren't we supposed to know ourselves, just from living with ourselves day in and day out, year after year? In truth, if we don't reflect and take time to get to know ourselves, we can stay very much in the dark. After more than fifty years, I am still shocked at how little I know myself sometimes. Just when I think I know who I am, I change. Half the battle is to know what I truly want, so I can give it to myself!

I've discovered that being self-aware is a great gift to give others. When I know and communicate what I need and what works or doesn't work for me, I give other people clear guidelines. They don't have to read my mind in order to avoid stepping on my toes. Conversely, my lack of self-awareness creates difficulties in my relationships. For example, I've had experiences traveling with a friend when I didn't realize that I needed some alone time or quiet time each day. If that did not happen, I found myself becoming irritable without knowing why.

Looking at myself through the compassionate eyes of the Witness, I can see that I need a lot of help. Yet I also see that this is true of most of us, and I'm neither ashamed nor sad about it. Nor am I proud of it. It's just the way things are.

The most powerful way to cultivate the Witness is through the practice of meditation. Sitting quietly, we observe our thoughts and feelings with acceptance, without judging or attempting to control or change anything. "Nonattachment" is a term used to describe a calm attitude toward thoughts and feelings, and ultimately toward whatever life brings. By not identifying with our viewpoints, opinions, or judgments, we begin to gain freedom from them. This is very different from refusing to look at or know about uncomfortable inner processes.

"Mindfulness" refers to the ability to go about our daily activities—breathing, walking, driving, speaking, eating—while being fully present and aware. This concept, which I first learned about in Thich Nhat Hanh's wonderful book *The*

Miracle of Mindfulness, sounds deceptively simple. The trouble is that our lives seem terribly complex. It's only possible for me to eat mindfully if I slow down, stop trying to read or listen to the radio or carry on a conversation at the same time, and put my full attention on each mouthful of food. Is it worth it? Whenever I eat with true mindfulness, I wonder whether eating disorders would exist if everyone simply practiced mindful eating. We would really taste our food, and we would be more in touch with our bodies to know whether the food was agreeing with us or not; we might know when we were eating to try to fill an emotional emptiness, and when we'd had enough.

Our breath is one of the greatest allies in the practice of mindfulness. Coming back to an awareness of breath, several times a day, is a deep practice of being present in the body, present in each moment. It's a wonderful refuge from the fears of the future and the regrets of the past. During these moments my Witness gains strength.

SPEND A LITTLE TIME EACH DAY reviewing your experiences while you are calm and relaxed, not giving more time or energy to what went badly or well, but just seeing it all from the slightly more distant perspective that time can give. It's very tempting to evaluate: "I did a great job on this, I did that terribly." Instead, simply look at it all and ask, "What can I learn about life? What can I learn about myself?"

The Inner Family

Practice hospitality to the differences within the self.
                                                    —John O'Donohue

In addition to our Inner Guide, Inner Critic, and Impartial Witness, we have an Inner Child, Baby, a rebellious Teen, and an Inner Adult or Parent. In my inner family, the Baby sometimes gets her way because otherwise she cries or is crabby and makes it hard for anyone else to have a good time.

When my Inner Child is happy, it's much easier to be generous and sweet to others. So, why am I not always good to her? Why not give her what she wants? Often, my Inner Adult/Parent judges her needs as selfish or unimportant, then tries to reason with her. When my Inner Adult decides to live in the present moment, without judgment and with gratitude and openness to whatever comes, new possibilities open up. The Inner Adult can then be compassionate and caring toward the Child, who becomes less complaining and demanding.

If I harm my Inner Child by not caring well for my body (lack of sleep, overwork, eating poorly), I get cranky. My Inner Child becomes irritable when her needs aren't being met. If I take better care of her, listen to her, and nurture her, I'm a lot happier. Instead of waiting for her to complain, it works best to plan fun activities that I know she'll like.

A few hours after a car accident, I realized that I had been feeling internally conflicted. A persuasive Chinese healer had talked me into signing up for a workshop in Palo Alto the next morning, and I was feeling exhausted. I was trying to cat-sit for a friend in Oakland, running back and forth to my apartment in Berkeley, and was overcommitted with various tasks. Although I was not injured, my car needed repair work, so I was unable to drive it to the workshop. If I had honestly and compassionately consulted my inner family, I would probably have realized that I didn't really want to drive to Palo Alto, and might have saved myself the trauma and expense of the accident.

If conflict reigns within the Inner Family, the Inner Witness can be a neutral mirror of what is happening, helping to defuse the struggle. Or I can call upon my Inner Guide for some direction. Once, when I was feeling down, my Inner Guide advised me to do some volunteer work. The experience of giving helped me to feel good about myself. The Critic could not find fault, and my Inner Child became a lot happier. There is no sense of sacrifice; in fact, it becomes easier to give to myself after I've given to another.

According to Hal and Sidra Stone, authors of *Embracing Our Selves*, each of us has some "disowned selves": the aspects of our personalities that we dislike, reject, or try to distance from. These aspects are not always negative. For example, a person raised by highly intellectual parents may have a disowned artistic self, such as a dancer or musician, if the parents discouraged the development of these talents. The disowned selves are kept from the light of conscious awareness, and hence become part of what Jung called our shadow. What we don't know, we fear. And yet this shadow may include our greatest source of creativity. We also tend to attract people into our lives who mirror the qualities that we have rejected in ourselves. They give us an opportunity to understand and accept those unloved aspects of our selves. More often, though, we will judge and distance ourselves from such people. I know a man who is so aware of his shadow's power that whenever he meets someone he dislikes, he makes a point of spending time with that person to see what he can learn.

For genuine integration and wholeness, I need to invite my disowned selves into the living room and get to know them. They just want to be heard and acknowledged; each has a valuable contribution. True self-love consists of embracing all aspects of the self.

TRY COMPLETING THIS SENTENCE: "I'm the kind of person who _has a strong Inner Critic._"

Gratitude

*Everything is gratuitous, everything is gift. The degree to
which we are awake to this truth is the measure of our
gratefulness. And gratefulness is the measure of our aliveness.* —Brother David Steindl-Rast

According to Neale Donald Walsch, author of *Conversations with God*, "Praying prayers of supplication is
not nearly as effective as praying prayers of thanks."
Even a little gratitude can have a most transformative effect.
When I feel grateful, I have a much fuller experience of whatever I'm appreciating, whether it is a sunset, an apple, or a
teaching; gratitude brings more of me into the present
moment. When I acknowledge a teacher and think about
something of value I've learned, the teaching becomes more a
part of me. When I see everything as a gift, nothing is really my
possession; hence, all is to be shared.

Native American teacher ChoQosh Au-Ho-Oh says that
when the sweat lodge feels too hot to bear, she reaches forward and welcomes the hot steam, brings it to herself, and
says, "Thank you." This makes her more capable of bearing
the heat. Caroline Myss recommends that we practice gratitude when feeling overwhelmed, and that we experience our
gratefulness to each person for the role he or she has played
in our lives.

At times it is difficult to see the gift in a situation. Remember those puzzle-pictures in which the fun was finding the hidden images? When I don't take the time to find the gift, I've just thrown away an offer of help extended by the universe. As in a treasure hunt, we are given only one clue at a time.

One day I was driving up to Mount Tamalpais for a solo hike, and on the radio was Mendelssohn's violin concerto—a favorite of mine. As I pulled into the parking area at the trailhead, I turned off the ignition but left the key in so I could hear the final notes of the music, which concluded just as I finished lacing up my hiking boots. The timing felt so perfect. As I picked up my daypack and shut the car door, I actually said "Thank you," to no one in particular, just for that perfection of timing. Suddenly, I realized that I had just locked my keys in the ignition! For a few seconds, my Inner Critic ranted: "You stupid idiot, you've locked your keys in the car AGAIN and you're nowhere near a phone, way up here on this mountain!"

Then I stopped. I had just said "thank you." What could I be thankful for? I realized that I was being given an opportunity to step away from my habitual pattern of self-blame and instead to practice trust. I could let go of my fearful need to control outcomes. Then and there, I made a commitment to myself that I would not call myself "stupid" because of this incident—not to myself, or to the person who would give me a ride to the telephone, or to the AAA driver who would come to unlock my car. I honored those commitments and I was given a ride by practically the first driver to come along. I had only a short wait for AAA. What I gained was the breaking of a very entrenched old pattern.

Criticism and complaining cause me to contract, whether I'm on the giving or receiving end. The habit of criticizing has even been said to cause arthritis. Gratitude, or appreciation, helps me to expand. The more I can appreciate—people, trees, flowers, birds, animals, sky, ocean—the more I expand. Silently blessing everything and everyone I meet can bring me great joy. Cursing is the opposite of blessing. How many times a day are you cursing what goes wrong, and thus sending energy into it? What would happen if instead you blessed what went well?

Some of the most emotionally mature people I know are people who have arrived at a place of gratitude for their parents. They came to understand and acknowledge the role their parents played in bringing forth the fullest expression of who they were. For example, I know a woman whose mother seemed to offer no support at all, even to oppose what her daughter wanted to become. However, since the little girl had a rebellious nature, her mother's opposition was the strongest possible incentive to go forward. Instead of saying, "I struggled hard to become who I am, against all the obstacles my mother placed in my path," this woman said, "If it were not for my mother's steadfast opposition, I might never have had such an intense motivation to pursue this career. She was the perfect parent for me."

We each have our unique ways in which we receive a little tap on the shoulder from the Universe. For me, when something arrives printed on yellow or goldenrod paper, I've noticed that it is often a special gift.

Stephen Levine, in his wonderful book *A Year to Live*, calls gratitude "the alchemist's secret," which "turns hell to heaven." He offers a meditation that includes this thought: "View the body with gratitude and the appreciation we might have for a simple old vase in which we daily find new flower arrangements."

When faced with a life-threatening illness, the most ordinary moments of life become extremely precious. A volunteer I met through the AIDS Project of the East Bay had recovered quite unexpectedly from what doctors had thought was a fatal brain tumor. Only a slight irregularity of his facial expression hinted at his previous illness. He recalled vividly how, as he lay in a hospital bed, not knowing whether he would live or die, his friends would come to see him. One of them complained about the traffic, snarled by a rainstorm. He lay there, thinking: "Oh, to be in that traffic jam. Oh, to be in that rainstorm!" At that moment, those everyday "nuisances" represented, to this young man, the richness of being alive.

YOU MAY WISH TO TRY THIS EXERCISE IN GRATITUDE: For one full day, look upon everything as a gift. Write about your experience, paying attention to the small details: the comfort of a cup of warm tea settling into your stomach; the beauty and perfection of sun shining through a green leaf.

Appreciate all the parts of yourself that are healthy, and all aspects of your life that work well, and you'll attract more of the same.

> *Everything is from Spirit.*
> *Everything from Spirit is a gift.*
> *Therefore, everything is a gift from Spirit.*

Judgments

*Everything in the universe has a purpose. There are no
misfits, there are no freaks, there are no accidents. There
are only things we don't understand.* —Marlo Morgan

Louisa's Wisdom

This chapter grew from many conversations with my
mother, Louisa Howe, who made a lot of progress in
her lifetime with overcoming judgmentalism. As a
teenager, she was belittled by her father, who frequently told
her, "You'll never be the woman your mother was." He had
such a low opinion of her that when she was accepted to Radcliffe College, he wrote to ask if there had been a mistake. She
went on to earn a Ph.D. in sociology. She became a staunch
defender of social justice and civil rights. Her expert testimony
was considered by some to be pivotal in the Brown vs. Board of
Education ruling on school desegregation.

She was by no means a perfect mother, but she kept working
on herself and growing. At age sixty she became a psychomo-
tor therapist. She often played the role of "ideal mother" for
her patients, and in many ways she became that. And yet, in
her final months of life she revealed the extent to which she
still judged herself quite harshly. "I'm failing," she would say,
hanging her head—as if weak vision and impaired hearing
were personal failures, or as if an unreliable memory made her

a worthless person.

My mother once told me a story about a drug-treatment halfway house where she had worked. One of the rules she established for the place was: "No labeling another person as right or wrong." Many times the residents would object: "But how can you help somebody if you can't tell them they're wrong?" Perhaps a more useful question is, how can you help people if you are telling them they're wrong? She saw that when people are loved and accepted as they are, they tend to grow and blossom. When people are criticized, they tend to resist change. Giving attention to "what's wrong" causes it to persist.

Blaming and shaming are two of the most damaging things we humans do to each other, she believed. "Praise is just the flip side of criticism," she would say, pointing out how praise is an evaluation and is often used to manipulate people. It is a strong discipline to avoid all evaluative words. Instead of saying, "excellent, great, beautiful, wonderful, well-done," notice how the other person responds when you say, "I appreciate, I like, it delights me, it touches me, I love . . . . "

NOTICE: How do you feel inside, when told you're wrong? Do you feel motivated to change, or to defend yourself?

How do you feel when someone praises you? Is there uneasiness?

Roots of Judgmentalism

Early on we are taught the importance of being "good," and "knowing right from wrong." When our parents don't like our behavior, they tell us we are "bad" or "naughty." When they approve of our behavior, we are "good" boys or girls. The child learns that being good equates with receiving love, while being bad means that love will be withheld. It becomes a matter of the child's very survival to be good, since otherwise he or she risks abandonment.

Parents often cloak their preferences in the language of moral imperatives to give more weight to their wishes and to evade personal responsibility for their likes and dislikes. Instead of "I don't like all that noise in the house," they say "It's wrong to make noise when Mommy is tired." Instead of "I want you to go to bed," a parent is likely to say, "Good children go to bed at eight o'clock." Use of terms like right and wrong, good and bad, have the effect of putting the burden of decision on some supposed external societal standard. Parents who do not feel secure with their own feelings about a child's behavior are more likely to call in an external standard instead of relying on their own authority and preferences. People who were taught to distrust or discount their own feelings have difficulty acknowledging those feelings when they become adults raising children.

Along with the right/wrong, good/bad labels come the imperatives of "should," "ought," "must," "have to." What must one do to be judged as good? What should one avoid doing to prevent condemnation? When parents teach children that they must be good in order to be loved, that is conditional love.

Of course, children need to understand the consequences of

their actions, such as that pulling the cat's tail hurts the cat or that running into the street is risky. However, these things can be communicated without the use of terms like "good" and "bad." It is more helpful for the child to feel empathy with the cat, to see tail-pulling from the cat's point of view, than to feel guilty and fear punishment for wrong-doing. Perhaps the limit-testing all children engage in comes from the very human desire to know at first hand the effects and consequences of their behavior. In this testing of limits, they are not only waiting to see if their parents will punish them; they are observing the emotions and responses of those affected by their actions. Hence, the importance of parents' expressing their honest emotional responses to their children's behavior: "I feel angry when you hit me," or "I feel upset when you throw your food on the floor."

Since most of what is presented to us as moral absolutes by parents and other authority figures is based upon their preferences, not everyone is raised to follow the same imperatives. For example, in one family, love may be bestowed upon the high achiever and withheld from the child who does poorly in school; while in another family, the "shoulds" are attached to being obedient and never talking back or showing anger. Inevitably, clashes occur between people brought up in families with differing value systems. A path away from conflict lies in the practice of unconditional positive regard and respect for all, regardless of their values, beliefs, or behavior.

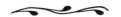

Nonjudging Language

Notice the effect of what you are saying to yourself and others. My mother would wince when anyone used the word "deserve," because she perceived it as laden with judgments about worthiness and unworthiness. Do you hear yourself using the word "perfect" a lot? Are you a perfectionist, frequently disappointed in yourself or others?

My friend and colleague Erik Peper taught me about replacing self-judging statements such as "I should, I have to, I ought to" with positive self-acceptance and awareness of choices: "I choose to, I want to, I could, I might." When you hear yourself saying, "You should" to another person, try substituting "It would please me if you would _____," or "I would like _____." Instead of "You should see this movie," try "You might enjoy this movie." Such phrases decrease the listener's defensiveness and increase receptiveness precisely because they are not moral imperatives, labels, or judgments of the other's behavior.

Instead of "I always do such and such," I'm learning to say: "At this moment in time, I do _____." This phrase opens the prison door by allowing me to change in the future. Also, I can trade "I can't" for "I haven't learned how—YET." Rachel Naomi Remen speaks of "the golden Yet," which represents the possibility of future growth and change.

Marshall Rosenberg, author of *Nonviolent Communication: A Language of Compassion*, believes that judging people is a suicidal way of trying to get our needs met. He recommends that we use descriptive language that is as neutral as a videocamera when referring to another's behavior. This takes some practice! For example, "When you yell at me" is not a neutral description. "When you raise your voice above mine" is much less loaded. After describing the behavior, we can communicate how we feel about it, again using nonjudging language. Stick with "angry," "sad," "afraid," and other direct descriptions of feelings. Avoid such terms as "betrayed," "abandoned," and "overlooked," which imply an interpretation of the other person's actions. After expressing our feelings, we can go on to communicating our needs and requests.

Lawrence LeShan, author of *Cancer as a Turning Point,* suggests a shift in focus from what's "wrong" with a person to what's "right." Instead of focusing on the disease, the focus for both healer and patient can become the life force seeking expression through creative endeavors or career. This has inspired me to ask clients about what they enjoy or appreciate rather than about their "complaints."

What I am saying to myself about a situation largely determines how I will react to it. If I call some work "drudgery," this is "judgery" that leads to "grudgery." My judgments of the work are harder for me to carry than the work itself. Exaggeration may generate exactly the opposite of what I really want. If I say, "I'm swamped," I'll feel more overwhelmed than if I say, "I'm very busy right now."

TRY OUT THESE PHRASES:
"At this moment in time" in place of "always"
"I choose to" instead of "I have to"
"I haven't yet" instead of "I never."

The Two-Edged Sword

We may be destroying our own self-esteem with harsh self-judgments, and then trying to bolster it again by judging other people. The habit of judgment-making is a two-edged sword incapable of being used only against oneself and not against others (or vice versa). Instead of saying to myself, "I did that wrong," I'm practicing saying "I'm not happy with how I did that," or "Next time I'll do that in a way that pleases me." I'm noticing that self-criticism comes from fear, and does not motivate me to change; it is more likely to make me want to defend my behavior. Similarly, my criticisms of others do not help them change, but cause them to dig their heels in and resist. By directing my energy into aspects I don't like, I actually cause those aspects to increase. True change is much more likely when I praise or appreciate, and thus reinforce, the desired behavior.

Safety seems to lie in finding a position of superiority from which to look down and judge others; however, the opposite is true, since no one exists outside a social context. The more we judge, the more we threaten our connectedness with others. Next time you're feeling judgmental toward someone, notice what happens to your ability to communicate with him or her.

When I was young, I discovered that I could defend myself from others' criticisms by judging myself before someone else could (or more harshly than anyone else would). Many of us are our own nastiest critics. Fear of our own self-condemnation is probably one of the most enduring fears. When, instead, we see ourselves as mirrored in the other, we can join and feel much greater love and safety than is ever possible in isolation and opposition.

On a recent Vision Quest, I asked a bird to teach me about

self-acceptance. At first it sat very still, and then it performed a 180-degree flip. This signified to me the need to make a complete turnabout in my way of seeing myself and others, from critical to compassionate.

When we become aware of how many times a day we are making mental judgments of ourselves or others, and begin substituting statements of unconditional acceptance, the results can be profoundly healing. Accept people as they are, and you'll have a thousand friends.

Judgments are the defense that I believed I needed, to keep my self intact and protect myself from disintegrating in times of stress. In reality, judging and comparing and blaming have been the greatest source of misery in my life.

Fight or Flight, Wrong or Right

When we judge another person, we feel angry or righteously indignant (ready for "fight"); when we judge ourselves or feel judged by others, we feel fearful and anxious (ready for "flight"). The fight or flight response is the body's way of responding to stress, and regardless of whether the threat is from within or from outside, the response is similar: the heart rate increases, blood pressure goes up, blood vessels constrict, breathing becomes shallow, muscles tighten, blood sugar and fat levels rise, the immune system and digestive system are suppressed. Repeated evocation of this response is an important factor in the development of disease—not to mention panic attacks, generalized anxiety, irritability, and depression.

Judgmental thinking generates defensiveness and concern about our status in comparison with others. Experts on heart disease describe the coronary-prone behavior pattern, which is based upon suspicion, distrust, hostility, and insecurity of status. Belief in scarcity usually accompanies and underlies this pattern. The perception that love and approval are scarce, since they were withheld by parents or granted only conditionally, results in the habit of withholding love and approval from oneself. The belief is that one must work harder and harder to earn love from self and others. One may also believe that time is scarce and that slow-moving or uncooperative people are in the way. The universe in general may be seen as a stingy place in which we must compete ruthlessly, in a zero-sum, winner-take-all game. "My gain is your loss, and vice versa. If you are worse, I am better, so it is in my interest to put you down." These beliefs and their resulting behavior patterns lead to stress and illness. Our highest priority needs to be the opening of our hearts.

Embracing the Shadow

When an inner situation is not made conscious, it appears
outside as fate.   —Carl Jung

Jungian psychology has emphasized the importance of the shadow: the disowned parts of ourselves that we project upon others, toward whom we then experience moral outrage or righteous indignation. Projection happens within our very closest relationships, as well as onto other groups like racial or religious minorities. Thus we see the phenomenon of "gay-bashing" by macho-men who deny their attraction to other men in fear of becoming homosexuals. Communists become the "evil empire." Complete self-acceptance seems to be the key to ending projection, whether onto one's spouse, a minority group, or another nation.

Many spiritual teachers have advised us that the shortest route to liberation and to peace in both the inner and outer worlds is to deal with our shadow. I had a dream once in which I met a woman who was both a victim and an abuser, and I knew that she was too much of a handful for me. I turned her over to a therapist friend, who called her whole extended family in for a session. This dream reminded me that the victim/abuser part of myself needs to be integrated with all my other "selves."

A profound shift in my level of honesty occurred one day when I suddenly saw how I became angry at my husband for mirroring back my judgmental perceptions of a friend. I was seeing my own shadow reflected, and I didn't like it at all—at first I tried to disown that judgment, and self-righteously pounced upon my husband for being so negative! However, I caught myself and said, "Let me try that again. It looks like you're mirroring back to me my judgments of our friend. I reacted and projected those judgments onto you! Now I see that you were just trying to join me in my perception."

Is your shadow looming large? Perhaps it's because you have been getting closer to the light.

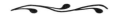

WHAT DO YOU JUDGE IN OTHERS? Is it the same as what you judge in yourself?

The Illogical Emotion

It's easy to say "love others, stop judging, open your heart." Learning to do these things is more challenging. A first step is to understand that we need no reason to love. Love, beauty, wisdom, hope, and faith are not logical; they are powerful forces in the universe, while logic is only a mental tool. If I wait for a rational reason to love another person whom I have defined as enemy, I'll be waiting a long time. When I love my enemy, he or she will no longer be my enemy. What gets in the way of my opening my heart is precisely my judgments, which come from the logical mind.

When I don't understand, my tendency is to judge. Now, I'm trying to remember to laugh instead. "I always laugh when I don't understand," says a young man in *Brother Sun, Sister Moon*, the film mentioned earlier about St. Francis of Assisi.

My friend Ria suggested to me that each time I catch myself judging someone, I stop and focus on seeing the good aspects of the person and then, find a way to make the person laugh! She practices this at the clinic where she works.

A shift in perception, in which I see that all people are doing the best they can, based on their beliefs and their past circumstances, can help me be more understanding. Forgiving and accepting myself is the basis for extending acceptance outwards. If I can forgive myself and realize that aggressive behavior is usually rooted in fear and pain, I can forgive the other person.

How do we expand our view? Travel and the study of many cultures provide an excellent way. Picture all the cultures of the world as a tall tower; each culture has a window facing in a slightly different direction. To get the full view of reality, we need to look through all of those windows.

IN THE BABEMBA TRIBE OF SOUTH AFRICA, when a person acts irresponsibly or unjustly, he is placed in the center of the village, alone and unfettered. All work ceases, and every man, woman and child in the village gathers in a large circle around the accused individual. Then each person in the tribe speaks to the accused, one at a time, about all the good things the person in the center has done in his lifetime. Every incident, every experience that can be recalled with any detail and accuracy is recounted. All his positive attributes, good deeds, strengths and kindnesses are recited carefully and at length. The tribal ceremony often lasts several days. At the end, the tribal circle is broken, a joyous celebration takes place, and the person is symbolically and literally welcomed back into the tribe.

A Dialogue with My Higher Self

Here are some excerpts from a written dialogue, inspired by Neale Donald Walsch's *Conversations with God*. I asked the questions, and my Higher Self answered them.

Q: How can I improve my self-esteem?

A: High self-esteem comes not from self-improvement but from letting go of false notions of who you are. It's only fear that makes you see yourself as limited: fear of failure and fear of others' reactions, such as envy.

Q: So I need to cope with my own envious and attacking responses to others?

A: Yes, and also practice trusting yourself, trusting God. When the impulse to attack and criticize yourself arises, observe it, comment on it if you like, but don't give in to it! Know it as a manifestation of fear. The more you criticize yourself, the more you'll criticize others. You'll be a lot happier when you stop.

Q: How does comparison keep me locked into low self-esteem?

A: Because you can always find someone who looks better than you!

Q: Well, duh! Why did I ever believe it was going to bolster my self-esteem?

A: When you compare yourself with others, you swing back and forth: better than, worse than. When you see yourself as better, you feel good for awhile. But people pick up on that air of superiority. They feel attacked, threatened, coerced. That's no good for relationships! Then you swing the other way, into self-doubt, self-attack, self-condemnation. That removes you from the guilt about superiority, but it's not viable either. *Stop all comparisons.* They keep you stuck in low self-esteem and toxic relationships.

Q: That seems so clear now. But it's such a deeply ingrained habit, I need some easy steps to follow.

A: Step number one: Take a good look at the past. How have comparisons and criticisms destroyed your relationships? Ask forgiveness, and seek to rebuild them through expressing appreciation. Even silent, or telepathic, appreciation can work!

Step number two: Offer service to others, as a means of feeling worthwhile. While you're in a serving relationship, your judgments tend to be on hold. You will focus on how you can help.

Step number three: Notice, with vigilance, mindfulness, and compassion, as the old habitual thinking reasserts itself. Decline to follow its bidding. This is the 180-degree shift you are being called to make.

We can all be way-showers and light-bearers for one another.

Another Way of Seeing

*The real voyage of discovery rests not in seeking new
landscapes, but in having new eyes.*   —Marcel Proust

One of my favorite fables illustrates the practical
importance of a shift in perception. It comes from a
James Thurber story my father read to me when I was
a kid, called *The White Deer*. In this off-beat fairy tale, each of
three princes is challenged with a series of tasks to win the fair
maiden. Prince Jorn, the youngest brother, must pick a thousand cherry-sized rubies from an enchanted cherry tree. He is
told by a small man in a peaked cap that he must count to one
thousand in order for each ruby to drop into his silver chalice.
He dutifully chants through the numbers, his hope of winning
the beloved lady steadily evaporating as time ticks by. The
small man starts questioning him: "Does a cherry drop when
you say ninety-nine?" "No," replies the prince. "Does a ruby
fall when you say nine hundred and ninety-nine?" continues
the man. "No," says Jorn. "When does a cherry or a ruby fall?"
"When I say one thousand," answers the prince. Just then, a
ruby falls into his chalice. "One thousand! One thousand! One
thousand!" cries Jorn, as the tree rapidly yields its enchanted
fruit in one-thousandth the time.

My five-year-old friend David reminds me of this principle
when he says, "One, two, skip a few, one thousand."

It is said that enlightenment can be attained by watching a

thousand sunrises and a thousand sunsets. Perhaps one sunrise would do, if I knew the magic words, or if I were simply fully present.

Einstein once said, "There are only two ways to live your life. One is as though nothing is a miracle. The other is as though everything is a miracle."

An exciting shift in perception came when I was in public health school and trying to secure a summer internship. Two of my classmates, also studying occupational health and safety, were interested in the same position I was angling for. After we had all been interviewed, the director advised us to settle it amongst ourselves, although she hinted to me that I had the most experience of the three. We had two weeks to make our decision. My classmates seemed ready to concede to me, but it didn't feel right. As I agonized about this to friends, most of them said, "Go for it, Cathy. It's your career!" But I realized that if I did, I'd feel guilty and my classmates might be resentful. Yet, if I magnanimously stepped aside, I could imagine one of my classmates looking guilty and myself feeling resentful. Back and forth I went in my mind between these two scenarios, thinking "There must be a better way!" I kept reminding myself of my values: placing friendship above career concerns, looking for win-win situations.

Then one day, like a stroke of grace, it came to me: There is no scarcity of learning opportunities! My dilemma had been based on the limited view that this one internship was the only place I could learn what I needed. With this insight, I felt as if the world had opened up again. My investigations yielded several promising internships, so I went to my classmates and announced that I now had other irons in the fire, and either of them could speak for the occupational health position. To my surprise, they each told me that they had found other internships. By letting go completely, I had been given back my original desire. Yet the biggest prize was my new learning: that when I drop my perception of scarcity, the world becomes a very abundant place.

When I lived in Boston, I was robbed a number of times in the 1970's, but the last time was unique. I had no car at the time, and was carrying a large bag of groceries down into the subway station. Having pulled out my wallet to purchase my fare, suddenly I realized the wallet was no longer in my hand. Turning, I caught a glimpse of a small boy who could not have been any older than six, whizzing up the stairs at lightning speed. After I got over the shock, I had to laugh, and even admit a bit of grudging admiration for his pluckiness. My view of myself as a robbery victim must have been permanently shifted by that experience, because I've never been robbed again to this day.

Seeing things with a different twist is the essence of humor. My father often attracts curious stares as he rakes up seaweed off the beach to use for mulching his garden. He loves to mutter, "I hate to see this mess, gotta clean it up." Sometimes he grins at people and says, "High fiber breakfast cereal."

Gentle eyes perceive a gentle world. A client whose vision was blurring due to multiple sclerosis. was about to lose her job as a result. Through developing awareness of her tension patterns with biofeedback, she was able to notice a correlation between harsh, judging thoughts and a hardening around her eyes. As she practiced softening her gaze upon the world and loosening the grip of her judgments of self and others, her vision gradually cleared up.

Am I focusing on the foreground or the background? One day I was visiting a friend who was dying of AIDS, in a room high up in Kaiser Hospital. Somehow I knew that this would be

the last time I would see him, and as I waited for the elevator
to take me back down to the lobby, I wept. In front of me there
was a window, smudged and scratched. As I looked at the window I thought how unfair it was that such a sweet young man
should die. Then I noticed that on the other side of that
window, the sun was setting in glorious shades of gold and
crimson. And I got the message. The choice is mine,
whether to focus on the ugliness in the foreground, or the
beauty in the larger view.

*We need a great rainbow in the soul to keep all the colors of
the light that we need for our vision.* —John O'Donohue

Transformation

Full fathom five thy father lies;
Of his bones are coral made;
These are pearls that were his eyes;
Nothing of him that doth fade
But doth suffer a sea-change
Into something rich and strange.
                                    —William Shakespeare

Even the times of deepest despair can be the cocoon-dark
prelude to a glorious rebirth.

The most astounding evidence I have found concerning
human beings' ability to transform comes from research done
by the Institute on Noetic Sciences on multiple personality disorders. We rarely think of the human body as fluid enough to
change in the twinkling of an eye; and yet, a person with multiple personalities may have diabetes in one personality and

not in another; may have disabling allergies in one, such as anaphylactic shock in response to orange juice, while in another personality he can drink it by the quart. Even an eyeglass prescription may be different from one personality to another. There is no way to explain this except that our bodies respond profoundly and immediately to our thoughts, feelings, and perspectives.

Language is a tool for changing our experience. When we refer to "the" pain instead of "my" pain, we can experience a sense of spaciousness; we are sharing in the human condition. We do not have to identify with the pain or illness, but can become much larger than it, with compassion for the suffering part of ourselves. Stephen Levine says, "When it's 'my' depression, 'my' cancer, 'my' AIDS, I am isolated from the source of my greatest comfort. But when it's 'the' depression, I take it less personally and am not too threatened to investigate it." Caroline Myss suggests becoming "the editor of your illness who can rephrase and delete those words from your mind, your heart, and your spirit."

How can we transform relationships? When I was teaching adult education courses, there was a certain secretary who used to give me a hard time. If my paperwork was late or not filled out correctly, she would scold me in a sarcastic, demeaning way, leaving me feeling humiliated. I began to dread going to the office. Finally I decided to create a shift in our relationship with a dramatic act: I ordered a dozen roses to be delivered to her, anonymously. I have no idea whether she ever figured out who gave them to her, but after that I no longer felt shame and dread in her presence.

Nature is constantly teaching me about shape-shifting. These visual metaphors point the way to a larger understanding of reality. A butterfly showed me how easy it is to disappear just by turning another aspect of itself to the viewer. Viewed head-on with its wings closed, it is almost invisible. Many creatures are able to blend in with their surroundings and disappear completely from our perception. In doing so they remind us that we are really not separate, but are shifting forms of one substance.

> *Lizard sits so still*
> *Blends with wood and becomes it.*
> *All beings are one.*

> *Little flat sandfish*
> *Disappearing perfectly*
> *Into ocean floor.*

> *Fish becoming sand*
> *At one with all surrounding,*
> *No separate self.*

> *Sun on spider silk:*
> *Cracks in reality's seams*
> *Show the light beyond.*

When we do the work of transformation, the inner and the outer worlds are often more related than we think. Once after clearing three large bagfuls of trash off a beach, I felt a giant boost in aliveness and kinship with the natural world. Restoring the Earth restores us as well.

A garden provides rich soil for transforming human beings. Cathrine Sneed, founder of The Garden Project at the San Francisco County Jail, describes the shift that occurs when inmates give away produce they've grown to kitchens feeding the homeless. The following testimonial comes from an article about the Garden Project in the Institute of Noetic Sciences's journal, *Connections:*

"When I was selling drugs," says a former prisoner who now works at the Garden Project, "I felt ugly inside and so I acted ugly in the outside world, but being in the garden and watching things grow has helped me to see the beauty in life. This is what the garden does. It ain't about growing spinach. It ain't about growing vegetables. It's about growing people."

Groundhog Day

Will the groundhog see his shadow? Will I step off the same curb into the same puddle? Or take a different street?

Will I live as if today mattered? As if this were the ONLY day of my life?

There is a wonderful, funny movie called *Groundhog Day* in which the cantankerous weatherman hero must live and relive one day of his life until he finally gets it right. I read in *The Boston Globe* this quote from Trevor Albert, the film's producer: "The Buddhists wrote saying they loved the movie and really appreciated the fact that it was made with a Buddhist philosophy. Then a couple of months later, Christian groups wrote saying they liked the Christian theology. And then the Jews wrote us, too." Even academics at European universities discuss it. It was named by Stanley Cavell in *The New York Times Magazine* as a "work created in the late 20th century that will still be discussed, viewed, and cherished 100 years from now."

Groundhog Day is the "cross-quarter holiday" that occurs on the second day of February, which is the midpoint between the winter solstice and the spring equinox. It was considered by the ancients to be the time when, deep within the dark and quiet soil, seeds begin to stir invisibly with the mysterious life force. It can be a time for contemplation, for reflection on that which we wish to create. In the Christian tradition it is called "Candlemas," celebrating the presentation of Christ in the temple; many candles are lit. In our contemporary folklore, the upcoming weather is determined by the groundhog: If he sees his shadow, there will be harsher winter weather ahead. The movie reminds us that our attitudes create our own inner "weather."

Life is like a board game. (Are you bored with the game?) Today is a new opportunity to wake up from the collective nightmare of repeated self-defeating patterns.

HOW WOULD YOU LIVE if this were the last day, or the only day, of your life?

Slowing Down and Waking Up

The soft breezes of the dawn have secrets to tell you.
Don't go back to sleep.   —Rumi

We shall not all sleep, but we shall all be changed.
                    —I Corinthians 15:21–22

Perhaps the time is at hand for the Great Awakening to occur. It doesn't feel as if we're asleep, but the great sages and mystics of many traditions have assured us that we are, that we are dreaming this nightmare illusion we call reality. When a nightmare gets too intense, my usual response is to wake up, with great relief. How bad must this nightmare get?

If life is really a dream, we might look deeply at the symbols that are showing up. What if we were to view our waking life as if it were a dream? What if everything were a communication to us, if we could only understand it? One day I saw a snail on the bed. Of course, I could rationalize that it was probably carried in from outdoors by our long-haired cat. Or I might see it as a broad hint to slow down. While at my mother's house trying to deal with all the physical clutter of magazines and mail and junk, which reminded me of my own mental clutter, I was feeling awfully serious and frustrated. Suddenly, out of nowhere, a pink helium balloon wafted into the yard—a reminder to lighten up?

The ability to choose consciously within a dream, which is referred to as "lucid dreaming," depends upon our knowing that we are asleep. It is the result of greater conscious awareness during the dream state. On those rare occasions when I have had a lucid dream, I have chosen to fly. The excitement and joy of knowing I am choosing my dream usually wake me up quickly! Perhaps the next stage in our evolution, before waking up completely, will be to choose our dreams.

The Andean shamans believe that humans have dreamed the current pollution and destruction of the Earth into being. They call upon humanity to change to an Earth-honoring dream, to bring healing to our planet. The images we carry reveal our intentions, and hold subtle power. We must be able to envision the change we wish to see. Perhaps when the collective dream shifts from "get rich quick" to "live in harmony," our actions will change accordingly.

Various forms of anesthesia are widely available these days. Alcohol, drug abuse, overeating, shopping, workaholism are all ways of numbing the pain of existence. What will rouse humanity from our dream-like state of unconsciousness about the devastating effects our lifestyle is having upon the planet? Reports of the extinction of thousands of species, cutting of the last old-growth forests, depletion of fisheries, serious loss of topsoil, pollution of air, water, and land, severe weather patterns caused by global warming, increased cancers and other environmentally caused diseases have not resulted in a decisive change of direction as yet. This is true even though it is becoming more and more clear that it is our own nest that we are fouling, our own children whose inheritance is being squandered. Many believe that a collapse of the current economic system is now inevitable.

Some folks believe that we are powerless to act, or that we can leave it to "the experts" to solve the messes we have created; yet there are no global agencies with the mission of protecting environments. Many feel that they just don't have time to deal with these huge issues of environmental destruction; they are already overwhelmed with trying to make ends meet and take care of their children. And so, we become numb. With the Y2K scare over, we are being lulled back to sleep by the siren songs of fossil fuel and technology.

Lack of time is cited as the reason for leaving children in the care of the TV set, eating prepared foods instead of home-cooked, failing to communicate fully with our loved ones, driving instead of bicycling, and not getting to know our neighbors. We hurry along, cell phones glued to our ears.

"Where evolution once described an interaction between humans and nature, evolution now takes place between humans and human artifacts," says Jerry Mander in his book *In the Absence of the Sacred*. "We coevolve with the environment we have created . . . . It's a kind of in-breeding that confirms that nature is irrelevant to us."

As the pace of life has become faster and faster, it seems impossible, even foolish, to slow down and take time to meditate or to just be, quietly in nature. Gandhi observed: "I have so much to do today, I need to meditate twice as long." Being in too much of a hurry prevents us from being able to hear our inner guidance, and makes reverence impossible. According to Angeles Arrien, "We kill our dreams by being too busy."

We are always going so fast, rushing, rushing to get more things done in a shorter time. Our language reflects how we have made time into a commodity: "Time is money." We "spend" time. We have been taught that if we hurry now, we will have more time later. It is slowly dawning on me that this is an illusion, perhaps one of the biggest illusions of the modern age. Speed has become a god. Labor-saving devices are embraced unquestioningly, since they are supposed to give us "more leisure time," and yet, the more technology we have, the more rushed our lives are becoming. Perhaps by worshiping speed, we become imbued with its energy, and unable to slow down. Speed breeds speed. And the faster we go, the more unconscious we remain.

We cannot be mindful of our actions or thoughts when we are in a rush. When we are driving fast, it occupies all of our attention to make sure we don't have an accident or miss our turnoff; there is scarcely any attention left for noticing the environment, perceiving beauty or uniqueness, or examining our thoughts. There are so many times when I was hurrying, then forgot something very important and had to go back for it, using much more time than if I had been more deliberate and thoughtful of what I was doing. And yet I stubbornly resist slowing down. It's partly because I place such a high value on productivity, after many years of being judged (and judging myself) on the basis of my achievements.

Acceleration creates anxiety, and harms relationships among people, by making us impatient with each other. If people are not going fast enough to suit me, I start to see them as obstacles in my path. If I am not giving myself enough quiet time and breathing space, I cannot give it to anyone else. My impatience with myself is transferred onto everyone I encounter.

Once, when I was rushing to a meeting, I failed to see a "Yield" sign. My peripheral vision did not seem to be working. Next thing I knew I was in a collision with another car. Luckily, no one was hurt, but I was left with a damaged car. I had received a not-too-subtle reminder that I need to do less charging straight ahead, and more slowing down, opening up my wider vision and "yielding."

As Caroline Casey said on her radio program *The Visionary Activist*, "When we learn to slow down, we won't need to hire authority figures to give us speeding tickets."

If we are always in a rush, there is literally no time to feel our feelings. I suspect that this is one of the hidden seductive aspects of being busy. We leave ourselves no time to feel grief over a loss, regret over an injury we've caused, pain over a rejection. It was very important for me to attend a grief support group after my mother's death, and at each meeting I experienced the bittersweet sadness of my loss. Yet, between meetings, it was easy for me to become so engrossed with my own busy life that I was unaware of my grief. Without the support group, I might have simply pushed away the feelings, deferring or refusing to feel them. I encourage anyone who has suffered a loss to take the time to be with those feelings—even if you think you are finished with them.

Compared with human time, Earth time is much slower. What is one human lifetime next to the life history of our planet?

When I give myself some time in nature, my frenzied urban rhythm shifts into lower gear. My breathing and heartbeat become slower, more relaxed. Sometimes I become aware how unnatural it is to consume caffeine and sugar, which speed me up more. Lately there have been reports that the Earth's vibrational frequency is quickening. Is the frantic pace of humans causing the Earth's frequency to increase?

In Buddhist mindfulness practice, one eats very slowly, chewing each bite of food twenty times or more, really tasting it, and receiving the gifts of the sun, rain, earth, and the toil of human hands that made the food possible. Eating in this way is an incredibly sensuous experience, and I notice that I don't need to eat as much in order to feel very satisfied. Mindful walking involves awareness of the breath, the surroundings, the weight being placed on each foot, and the thoughts: it enables us to be fully present in each moment.

Optimism and pessimism both reflect attachment to future outcomes. Neither attitude is focused on the present moment, where life is to be lived. Those who do the most outstanding service are often those who act from love, without expectation or attachment to the results of their efforts. Dick Roy, founder of the NorthWest Earth Institute and tireless volunteer for the Earth, recommends "viewing optimism and pessimism as distractions."

The Buddhist concept of awakening refers to being fully conscious, fully aware. In an oft-quoted story of the Buddha, he is asked, "Are you a god? An angel?" To which he responds, "No, I am awake."

Waking up is hard to do! Sometimes it even feels like breaking up. Who has not had the experience of shutting off the alarm clock and going back to sleep? A friend of mine says we are all here to help each other awaken, but often our response to those well-meant attempts to rouse us is grumpiness, insults, or hurled pillows. The true friend continues trying despite all our complaints. When we finally awaken, we are very grateful for the persistent, loving nudges that prevented us from being late for an important commitment. But while we are still snoozing, the friend's behavior seems most irksome.

The best way to make our dreams come true is to wake up.

Perhaps we've been "half-brained" (using only the left brain) for too many years and the time has come to reawaken the nondominant hemisphere. Our best rational, logical and scientific thinking got us into this mess. Practices of reverence, humility, meditation, prayer, ritual, and listening for guidance in sacred time were largely put aside while we marched to the beat of technology. To live in balance with nature, we need to slow back down to nature's rhythm, walking instead of driving or taking jet planes. In the history of humankind's life on Earth, only certain indigenous peoples, whose notion of time was circular instead of linear, lived sustainably. Their way of life is gravely threatened by our all-consuming culture. What can we learn from them that might apply to our present situation?

HERE ARE SOME PRINCIPLES:

- When planning, take into account the effect of our actions on the seventh generation from now. Doing something for the coming generations is not self-sacrifice! Most businesses fail to look past the next six months.
- Sitting in councils, bring forth the wisdom of the circle for making important decisions.
- Live with respect for, and in harmony with, other species—not as if ours were the only one that mattered.

Many indigenous cultures perceive spirit as dwelling in all aspects of the natural world.

- Seek fulfillment through connection, rather than through acquisition.
- Balance giving with receiving; offer thanks for what is received.
- Ask for spiritual guidance and support.
- Align with the natural cycles of the seasons, of night and day, growth and decay.
- Perform rituals of honoring the more-than-human forces and rituals of atonement when we have done harm.
- Take action to restore what was damaged.

These ways of life arise from, as well as generate, awareness and reverence for the Spirit in all of creation. May we all awaken to such an awareness, through slowing down enough to touch and feel it.

No Victims, Only Volunteers

*Your grief for what you've lost lifts a mirror to where you
are so bravely working.*   —Rumi

*There is no such thing as a problem that does not have a gift in it.
If you have many problems, it is because you need many gifts.*
                                          —A *Course in Miracles*

Time Out

When we see ourselves as victims of some injustice,
unhappy and powerless, the consolation prize is
that we can feel righteous. We imagine that being
right will make us happy, but the truth is that we can choose to
be happy and not be victims.

One quick way I've found to choose happiness is to start
appreciating something in another person, or in my own situation. I'm also experimenting with the idea of "choosing to
take risks." Risks find us anyway, so maybe I can get one-
up by pretending to choose the risks—or even by really
choosing them.

The most arresting examples of people who refuse to see
themselves as victims come from concentration camps. In his
classic, *Man's Search for Meaning,* Victor Frankl wrote:

We who lived in concentration camps can remember the men who walked through the huts comforting others, giving away their last piece of bread
. . . They offer sufficient proof that everything can
be taken from a man but one thing: the last of the
human freedoms—to choose one's attitude in any
given set of circumstances, to choose one's own
way.

I'm so lucky. I received a sabbatical: several months off work,
with pay, to study, play, get wiser, heal myself, and write. Or I
could say that I received several months off work, with pay, to
study, play, get wiser, heal myself, and write. Before you turn
green with envy, wait a minute. Are you out of work because
of illness or injury? Or were you laid off from your job, as I was?
Then, you're lucky too. You also have been given a sabbatical.

What's a sabbatical? It's a time of rest, like the Sabbath. This
implies that resting from one's labors and everyday pursuits has
a spiritual quality about it, and it does. It offers time for reflection and redirecting ourselves, even time for cultivation of our
souls. Our practice of keeping the stores open on Sundays
makes us poorer as a society. Business continues as usual, with
no slowing down.

I admit that being laid off, with unemployment benefits, is a
lot easier to deal with than being seriously injured or ill. But
that didn't stop me from seeing my situation through victim's
eyes for about eight hours: "Oh no—Just when I thought I had
a secure job and benefits, here we go again. Good hours, good
pay, nice people to work with—no more. What will become of
me? I'm fifty years old!" The tears flowed. Once the victim perspective was in place, next came the voices of self-doubt. My
Inner Critic sneered, "If you were more skilled in your work,

this wouldn't have happened. You didn't put out enough effort or promote your services enough." Insincerely, I affirmed: "I'm sure something good will come out of this," and "When one door closes, another one opens."

Then it dawned on me. I was free! I could do just about anything I wanted to do with my time and still have a modest income. As soon as this awesome fact came home to me, all thoughts of victimhood vanished.

Some folks who have become ill or injured realize later that it was a gift. They see that what they most needed at that time in their lives was time off from the pressure and routine of work, to contemplate, rest, and redirect their lives. Others unfortunately stay stuck in feeling like victims. Perhaps this comes from the ingrained fear of being judged for being "unproductive"—as if earning a paycheck were the only worthwhile use of our lives. So, to justify this time of "nonproductivity," people identify with the victim role: "It happened to me, I didn't want this." As Brother David Steindl-Rast reminds us, whatever life gives us is a "given," so why not regard it as a gift?

Dr. Christiane Northrup says, "Illness is often the only socially acceptable form of Western meditation." Our society does not recognize the universal human need for rest and reflective time.

My friend Ria told me that when she broke her elbow, although it was quite painful, the time off which it gave her was a true gift. "I planned my whole garden in my mind. I went door to door on my street and organized my neighborhood to get a speed bump."

Often the biggest obstacle to healing is our self-identification as victims. Labeling ourselves as victims effectively drains away our potential healing power. It sends a message of helplessness to the inner self, and to the very cells of our immune system, so of course there is less energy available for healing.

Caroline Casey, radio talkshow host and author of *Making the Gods Work for You*, advises us that casting ourselves as victims in our stories is too costly. Instead, she suggests that we look at our childhoods as "research" that enables us to become wiser and more compassionate.

Which part of myself am I identifying with? If I don't act the part of the helpless child, there will be no room for the punishing parent in my life. Sometimes I confuse my hurt with the person I am, identifying only with the hurt and not with my strength. If I see my wound as a gift, then perhaps I won't need it anymore.

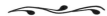

IF YOUR INJURY WERE AN OPPORTUNITY, what would it be inviting or freeing you to do (or not do)? What benefits does it confer?

Responsibility

What if your soul had chosen everything that happens to you, including all the problems and catastrophes and trials and illnesses, for the valuable lessons you could learn from them? Many people believe that we have reincarnated many times and that our actions in a previous life generate "bad karma" for which we must atone. Do you think you were a murderer in a previous life? According to the Buddhists, we have all done terrible things in one lifetime or another, but our present life problems are not a punishment for evil-doings. The Dalai Lama once observed, "Sickness is rarely karmic."

What is karma, anyway? It can be seen as cause and effect. If you throw an apple into the air, it comes down. Depending on how you throw it, it may come down on your head. We get to see the effects of our actions, that way, and hopefully learn something. If I hate my stomach for being "too big," my stomach may start to hurt after awhile. Cause and effect.

I always have a choice. I can say, "God is punishing me," and feel like a victim. Or I can say, "I don't know why I have this stomach ache. Maybe I can find out." Ask your stomach, "Why do you hurt?" It may say, "Because you're mean to me." Then you have another choice. You can start to be kinder to it, and observe what happens.

Often when illness or injury occurs, I look around for someone or something to blame: my boss for overworking me, myself for not listening to my body sooner, my family for making too many demands on me, my parents for raising me the wrong way—the list is endless. When I point the finger at someone, it's very easy to get stuck in blame and anger, which does not help me heal. Whether I blame myself, another person, the universe, or God, blaming seems to shut down the healing process.

Here is an excerpt about taking responsibility from a letter written by Miki Kashtan, a courageous friend who was struggling with lymphoma (a cancer of the lymph system):

> I am trying to be really rigorous about not blaming anything or anyone for any feeling that I have, taking full responsibility for my actions and beliefs and feelings. It is so hard, it feels like the hardest thing to be doing to really own my life and not have it be happening to me. It is so much easier to put it on events or other people not doing the right thing. Sometimes it feels really awful to hold on to my responsibility, and that in and of itself triggers the

despair to the max, because I repeatedly come up against the belief that I have not made any progress in my work on myself, that I may never heal. The extent to which I myself am the main choreographer of my life, including the difficulty in finding room for myself, is staggering. This is not to say that I am to blame—only that I make choices, many of which are based on past painful experiences, choices that reinforce the painful messages and renew them. And I can make other choices, at least I can grope my way toward them. And that process is excruciating: it's about not waiting for anyone to guess and give me what I want, and instead asking for it. It brings me face to face with me to a degree I have not before experienced, and I am seeing things I probably have chosen not to see before.

I salute Miki for her courage in confronting herself and taking responsibility for getting her own needs met, and indeed, responsibility for her entire life. This is a profound form of self healing. Perhaps it is even, as Stephen Levine might say, "the healing we took birth for."

Some Tibetan monks were taken as political prisoners and forced to live in unspeakable conditions, yet none of them suffered from post-traumatic stress disorder, a condition that is common for political prisoners. Why not? These monks firmly believed that they were burning up many years of karma through this experience. Thus, they were not perceiving themselves as victims, but rather viewing their circumstances as an opportunity for spiritual liberation.

When we change our perspective and view an injury or illness as an opportunity to change direction, there is no one to blame.

An occupational injury can be an initiation into a deeper realm of life, where you confront existential questions such as, "Why me?" "Why was I injured, when I was only doing my best and working hard to support my family?" "Why must I suffer, while those who are responsible for my injury are pain-free?" As your inquiry deepens, these questions might give way to, "Why did I stay so long on a job where I wasn't happy?"

Sometimes, people find it difficult to leave a work situation that is not fulfilling their higher purpose, or even a situation that is toxic or abusive. There are fears: "What if I can't find a better job? I don't have many skills. Then I won't be able to support my kids. It would be selfish to quit." Or, "I'm only four years away from retirement now. It would be foolish to leave early and decrease my benefits. Besides, who will hire me at my age?" Or, "It won't look good on my résumé to stay here less than two years." Under such circumstances, when neither we ourselves nor society seems to give us permission to make a change, sometimes the only legitimate "way out" is to become injured or sick. This allows us to keep our dignity and avoid guilt. "I worked so hard on that awful job that now I'm disabled. I did my best." "I would have stayed on another four years, but I got sick."

If we have a lot of anger at authority figures such as our parents and felt victimized by them, these feelings may be transferred onto a supervisor or boss. If we give away too much of our own power and responsibility for our lives to such people, we will feel powerless and helpless. But the problem isn't that "they did that to us." It's up to us to reclaim our own power and responsibility for how we choose to live our lives now. This is part of the process of maturing fully.

Creating guilt or reproach does not help the situation. When we feel powerless, our only way to extricate from an impossible situation may be a breakdown in health. The point is to reclaim that power in order to get well. If you knew that by being miraculously healed tomorrow, you would be placed right back into the same intolerable situation, you might have a hard time getting over your injury or illness. I've seen this many times in people with occupational injuries. The injury got them out of a position where they felt stressed, undervalued, used, abused, or discriminated against. One woman with repetitive strain injury in both arms, who felt she had suffered racial discrimination in her workplace, experienced a surge of pain in her arms each time she spoke about the injustice done to her.

Of course, everyone wants pain or illness to stop. But what steps are we willing to take to find or create work that is more suitable, that is in closer alignment with our heart's dream? We all long for work that expresses our uniqueness, uses our skills, and contributes to making the world a better place. Perhaps most of us feel unequipped to find that, especially if there are young mouths to feed at home. The challenge is to hold on stubbornly to our dreams and our sense of purpose. What our children need more than a materially comfortable life is a positive role model: a parent who will not be beaten down by the "shoulds" of society, but who reaches for meaning and fulfillment of life purpose. The value of this gift to our children is inestimable.

Lawrence LeShan, Bernie Siegel, Carl Simonton, and other outstanding health practitioners who work with cancer patients encourage people to perceive their illness as a "wake-up call" instead of a death sentence. Through experiencing cancer as a message from the body that something in one's life is out of balance and needs to be changed (such as the job, the self-image, or a relationship), the person is better able to rise to the challenge. By taking a courageous step and discarding the

dead-end job or the lifeless relationship and pursuing vigorously whatever brings the greatest sense of joy and aliveness, a
person can sometimes arouse the immune system and drive the
cancer into remission. The former patient often remarks, "My
illness was the best thing that ever happened to me. It forced
me to reflect, to stop living the life prescribed to me by others
and start living my own life."

At one of my workshops, a woman with breast cancer suddenly realized that she loved to sing, but had never given herself permission. She lit up with joy as she pictured herself
singing in front of a group of cancer survivors to encourage
them to follow their dreams.

Forgiveness

> *Forgiveness is the key to happiness.*
> —A *Course in Miracles*

Are we to blame for not having changed our lives sooner,
before the illness or injury? Are our families, teachers, or religious leaders to blame for having trained us to live our lives the
"wrong" way? I don't think so. We are all doing the best we
can, and we're all human and very fallible.

Healing can be incredibly swift when a person is in a state of
acceptance, love, and forgiveness. Forgiveness is not a denial
of pain, nor is it a condoning of what has happened. True forgiveness is the recognition that we all act unskillfully out of our
woundedness, and that holding onto resentment hurts us more.
To forgive is to transform anger into love.

At the San Francisco Whole Life Expo I once heard a man
tell the story of his remarkable recovery from a parachuting

accident. He emphasized that what seemed most important in his healing was that he did not blame himself or anyone else involved in the event. Also at the Expo, a few years later, I heard two men, Chris Loukas and Steve Backman, tell a remarkable story. Two years before, Steve was addicted to drugs and alcohol. He had been drinking, and his car hit Chris' in a 60 mph head-on crash. The doctors did not expect Chris to live; he was in a coma for six weeks. When he regained consciousness, he asked his family to seek out the other driver so he could extend heartfelt forgiveness. They had an emotional meeting in his hospital room. Afterwards, Chris' healing was very rapid. Steve entered recovery, and started upon a spiritual path. As Steve said, "The love from the Loukas family is better than any high!"

In ancient Hawaii, the kahunas (healers) had an interesting way of treating a sick person. The whole extended family would be summoned and each person was instructed to ask or offer forgiveness with anyone else in the family where it was needed. The process might take several days. When this amazing family systems therapy was completed, the sick person's health was usually restored.

Sometimes what we may need most of all is to forgive ourselves. "When I stopped judging myself, I realized that I wasn't guilty!" a friend confided in me. "No one else was judging me." As Brooke Medicine Eagle says, "Forgive yourself within, and you are forgiven."

Illness is a very complex matter. Great sages and saints have died of cancer. Tibetan Buddhists believe that some people contract illnesses because they have undertaken to carry some of the suffering of the world, to lessen the burden on others. Ultimately, we all die. When healing occurs on a spiritual level, it becomes less important whether or not the body heals.

HERE ARE SOME QUESTIONS to ask yourself:

- Where do I feel I've been treated unfairly?
- How has that perception influenced or changed my view of life?
- What fears did this belief give rise to?
- Whom do I need to forgive?
- What event from the past am I dwelling on; what would be necessary for me to resolve it?

Lively Work

*What is the meaning of your work? What does it symbol-
ize, stand for, or represent? This meaning is a powerful
predictor of life and death. We live out the meanings.
Meaning enters the body and makes the difference, in
many cases, in life and death.* —Larry Dossey, M.D.

*Our life is more than our work,
And our work is more than our job.*
—Charlie King

Our calling, according to theologian Frederick Buech-
ner, is the place where "our deep gladness and the
world's deep hunger meet." Many people believe that
we are born with a "soul purpose," some task that we feel
drawn to complete or a gift that we long to express. Discovering our life purpose and finding the courage to live it out is a
process that is unique to each individual. Some lucky ones
seem to have been born knowing their purpose and go straight
after it regardless of what their parents or teachers said. Most
of us need to stumble around a bit. Some people despair of ever
finding meaningful work; others hold back because they don't
feel qualified.

We look around and see a planet in trouble because too
many people have blindly done what seemed to be expected of
them, following the status quo, taking jobs that support the

consumer economy instead of doing what their hearts urge them to do. Now, more than ever before, the world needs the unique gift that each person has to give. And yet, it requires courage and patience to follow the path of the heart. Following that path may not provide an income right away, while we are developing our skills or getting the training we need.

According to Lawrence LeShan, who wrote *Cancer as a Turning Point,* many people with cancer have a history of having lost, or never found, their life's most important work; when assisted in finding or rediscovering it, a surprising percentage go into full remission. LeShan has a wonderful story about a New York City street-gang member whose buddies had all died or gone to jail. Languishing in a hospital bed with lymphoma, the young man felt that his life was over. LeShan drew out from his patient the key aspects of the gang lifestyle that were so fulfilling: crises calling for a strong team response, kick-back times of camaraderie. The life of a firefighter was similar enough to intrigue the former street fighter, and before long he was working toward his high-school GED. Years later, the young man was healthy, married, and enjoying his career.

Nor is cancer the only illness that occurs when we lose touch with our life's dream. In my years as a respiratory therapist, and later as a biofeedback therapist, I met many people whose illness or injury related to the lack of meaning they found in their jobs. A patient I met in the hospital was a severely asthmatic bus driver who also had a sleep disorder. He admitted that he hated his job, but was trying to stick with it for just five more years until retirement. When I asked him what he dreamed of doing instead of driving the bus, his face lit up and a new energy infused him. "I'd like to open my own little barbecue joint," he confessed. A young woman with a repetitive strain injury from her boring word processing job spoke longingly of a career as a radio personality.

No matter how desperate our circumstances, there is hope. After she fractured her spine and pelvis by leaping from the third story of a burning building, Ina Marx was told by doctors that she would never walk again. In the 1950's she was in constant pain, gaining more and more weight, addicted to prescription drugs and cigarettes. She attempted suicide twice. Then she discovered yoga, and regained her life. Teaching yoga became her passionate mission, and at age seventy she was slim and energetic, with the flexibility of a woman half her age.

Finding our soul's purpose is very much the hero's journey. However, unlike the solitary hero, we need not go it alone. Our path becomes clearer when we join with others in this quest. There's nothing like a support group for cheering each other on through the difficulties. Barbara Sher, author of *Wish-Craft,* suggests a brainstorming session or "Idea Party," where support group members invite their friends and come together creatively to solve the tough problems and share resources. The wildly unexpected and synchronous flow of spontaneous ideas makes this one of the most exciting and delightful activities I have experienced. People naturally enjoy assisting one another.

Balance is an important aspect of livelihood. For me, this means time working outdoors as well as indoors; having my hands in the soil as well as on a keyboard; learning as well as teaching; being with children as well as adults. What would bring more balance into *your* life?

Don't wait until you're perfect to begin doing the work you love. Start! An easy way to begin is by doing it as a volunteer. You may need to detach your self-worth from what you earn and how you earn it, since your highest value and biggest contribution might not come from your paid work. Our true worth does not depend on what we do; it is an unfortunate aspect of our culture that we are defined by what we do for an income. When our work feeds the soul and helps the planet, other things tend to fall into place.

Our work was meant to come from our hearts; our arms and hands were meant to give the gifts of the heart. One of my favorite prayers is "Use me!"

A shortcut to discovering your path and following your life's dream is to ask yourself these questions:

If I had only one year to live, what would my priorities be? How would I spend my time? What would I most want to contribute before I left? It is a great gift to know that death is certain but the timing is unknown. This awareness helps us to be present in the moment, rather than living our entire lives in the past or future.

Falling autumn leaves
Great beauty in letting go
Brightest colors come.

If I had just one year to live:

I'd start to follow my own advice. I'd think big, take more risks, and break more rules.

If it were my last spring, I'd spend more time admiring the flowering trees and daffodils.

I wouldn't take on any new karma; I'd work at clearing up all the old unfinished business.

Knowing that relationships are the most important aspect of life, I'd learn to communicate better and listen more.

I'd focus less on doing and accomplishing; when people inquired about my activities, I would mention my most outrageous and right-brained activities first, instead of the things I think they would approve of. I'd live radically, without fear of others' judgments.

I'd travel more, to gain perspective.

I would live the year as a giveaway, like a thundering waterfall, or like a bird singing *Gloria!*

I'd give myself the conditions I need to grow, including more play. Play is the key to happiness, power, abundance. With apologies to the Bard: Play's the thing with which I'll catch the consciousness of a King!

I'd live closer to nature.

I would focus on creating peace within me (acceptance of all parts of myself); peace between me and my family members, friends, coworkers, neighbors; peace between the human race and all other species ("all our relations"); peace on Earth.

Knowing that what dies is really my separate-self or ego, I am plotting its demise. Of course, if my ego is not dead by the end of the year, I can always get an extension on my misery.

If I had only a few months left to live, I'd hire people to do the things I'd rather not do.

And if I had just one day? I'd live it totally from my heart, with no excuses.

(By the way, if you received a certificate giving the date of your death, would you let me know how you came by it? Mine was missing; a shipping error, I believe.)

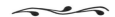

CONSIDER:

- What did you love to do as a child, aged nine to eleven?
- What activity did you lose yourself in, for hours at a time?
- What is your vision of a utopian society?
- What gift or talent would you be willing to share, to contribute to its creation?
- In your utopia, what would you be doing for the sheer love of it, whether or not you got paid?

Everybody has a gift to give to the world—so stop sitting on your assets.   —Swami Beyondananda

Nature

Nature as Teacher

*I think I could turn and live with animals, they are so
    placid and self-contain'd,
I stand and look at them long and long.
They do not sweat and whine about their condition,
They do not lie awake in the dark and weep for their sins,
They do not make me sick discussing their duty to God,
Not one is dissatisfied, not one is demented with the
    mania of owning things,
Not one kneels to another, nor to his kind that lived
    thousands of years ago,
Not one is respectable or unhappy over the whole earth.*
                                    —Walt Whitman

We humans have a tremendous amount to learn
from animals. They bring us back to our senses.
When they sit or lie down, they relax completely
every muscle they don't need. Watch especially the wild animals. Walk on an animal trail, such as bird tracks at the beach.
Imagine becoming that animal; try walking its walk. Hatha
Yoga has many postures that imitate animals and trees as a corrective for the way we live in our bodies as humans. These postures help us to align ourselves better with the natural world.

If you have ever done the "tree" pose indoors, try it while standing next to a tree and contemplating it. With bare feet, focus on sinking your roots deep into the ground. Even a back yard or city park can have trees and birds. Many standing yoga poses, done outdoors, help us open our hearts to the sun.

When we sit quietly in one place long enough, the wild creatures come around more. Birds come surprisingly close. I would love to be as inwardly quiet and clear as a certain Vision Quest guide I know, who has walked among a group of deer without alarming them.

Each natural entity that we approach with reverence and listen to, whether it be a bluejay, an oak tree, or a stream, can give us wondrous gifts. By deciding to be the student, I become able to learn. "You're my teacher. What can I learn from you today?" Nature mirrors to us parts of ourselves we didn't know.

Whatever humans have been saying to each other about animals, trees, stars—whether true or not—will be reflected back to us when we encounter that entity. If a large beetle appears in front of me, some of my early conditioning to despise all insects will show up, blocking my ability to be present and learn from it. On a subtler level, the lore about beetles as a symbol of resurrection, sacred to Egyptians, may be present in my mind as well. If I let go of what I think it means, I become more observant and the beetle can teach me more.

When I'm out in nature, I often focus on a problem or an issue I need some guidance about, then notice where my attention is drawn. Whatever attracts my eye or ear may be "calling" to me, perhaps with something of value to communicate. Am I willing to act on these messages? If my thoughts seem to stray away from what I am observing outwardly, I try to observe whether there was any correlation between that natural entity and the direction of the thoughts.

A stone can carry every bit as much meaning as a Tarot card or other human-devised divination tool. Once I picked up a reddish stone that caught my eye. As I examined it, I saw that it resembled an anatomical heart, even with faint lines suggesting the two atria and two ventricles. What I noticed was that the atria (which receive blood for the ventricles to pump out) were quite small, in proportion to the ventricles. This got me thinking: Is it hard for me to receive?

Once when I was pondering problems in my relationship, my attention was drawn to two birds who seemed to be a couple. They would fly together for a while, then go off in their separate directions, then rejoin. They seemed to be teaching me the wisdom of taking space, having frequent time apart.

One day when I was feeling a bit stuck, I perceived a smooth gliding movement. A snake flowed gracefully past me, heading downhill, staying completely in contact with the earth, then purposefully let itself drop down to the next level. As if to underscore what I was to learn, a second snake appeared and repeated the action. Each snake had showed me, in turn, how to stay grounded, yet let go and fall fluidly.

It seems that when an animal, bird, reptile, or insect guide shows up, I often receive the most benefit if I immediately follow or imitate the behavior it is showing me, as closely as I can with this human body. A lizard on a tree doing pushups inspired me to try a couple of modified ones; I noticed that it got me closer to the ground, which felt good, and also changed the level of my gaze, high-low-high-low. The lizard then became so still that I thought it had disappeared. Just as I was accepting that my teacher had gone away, it moved, and I realized what a magical shape-shifter this camouflaged lizard was. It was teaching me how stillness is a means of blending with and becoming the tree.

If my teacher is a tree, I enjoy standing next to it and looking out at the world from its viewpoint. What does it see, as it stands in one spot year after year?

A message I received from a waterfall: "If you are living life fully, you must constantly tear yourself away." Although it first struck me as a harsh message, I realized that losses are a natural part of life, and clinging to the past is not healthy.

Spiders and their webs fascinate me. A tiny gray spider visited me as I was writing in my spiral notebook, and amused itself by treating the loops of wire as a jungle gym, hopping from one to another. "Bravo," I said, admiringly, and the spider put its two front legs together as if applauding itself!

Once I noticed a miniature spider on one of my shoulders. Minutes later, it had crossed the continent of my back and was on the other shoulder. As if that was not enough of a feat, it then rappelled down from my head to dangle in front of my glasses. It's hard not to imagine that it was trying to get my attention.

The spider is not only an amazing trapeze artist and teacher of ropes courses, but also the creator of the original Web. I believe that after the Internet will come the Innernet, linking all minds. We'll move from telecommunication to telepathic communication when we remember that minds are joined. In Native American mythology, Grandmother Spider wove the web of connection that linked all of life.

One day as I sat by a creek, a ladybug was resting on my knee. When I stood up, the ladybug fell into a shallow pool in the creek and began struggling to swim back to dry land. Just as I was about to rescue it, I noticed two water striders moving toward the hapless ladybug. They made tiny waves as they jerked across the water, which helped wash the ladybug toward shore. What I saw next astonished me. One of the water striders placed itself between the ladybug and a leaf at the edge of the pool, forming a bridge. The ladybug was thus able to crawl onto the other insect's back and across its legs to the safety of the leaf. I am nominating the water strider for the Nobel Peace Prize for altruistic assistance to another species.

Our animal companions, who have adopted us as their pets, can be great teachers for us when we pay attention. Rainbow the cat (so named because as we were coming home with him in the car, a double rainbow appeared in the sky), tries very hard to teach me things. Frequently I am much too dense or preoccupied to get it, but one winter he astonished me by going up on the roof in the pouring rain. Normally cats avoid getting wet, but not this one. He meowed loudly for help, until I came out to rescue him. He has certainly never been one to play it safe. From him I learned: Take risks, no matter how uncomfortable it is, and holler for help until it comes.

Poetry helps break through the bounds of cultural constraint, whether between differing groups of people or between human culture and that of nature. Angeles Arrien and Michael Cohen showed me how effective haiku can be as a way of letting nature's message emerge.

> *Haiku mind and form:*
> *A human-sized opening*
> *That spirit comes through.*

Once as I was pondering my future, a tiny caterpillar captivated me with its boldness:

> *Small caterpillar*
> *Fearlessly bungee jumping*
> *Explores the limits.*

While walking a forest trail, notice any obstacles in the path. Our tendency is to focus so much on our destination that we regard obstacles as nuisances. Obstacles do get our attention, and so they deserve special observation. In what way is this obstacle representative of other kinds of obstructions, such as the ones we encounter on our path through life? Sketching a fallen log may reveal more than first meets the eye.

Sometimes the messages I receive are unexpectedly funny. One day when I was hiking I became unsure of which way was the trail to the waterfall. There was no signpost to guide me; or so it seemed at first. Taking a step back, I looked up and saw a dead tree whose branches were all broken off on one side. On its other side, at least eight branches were pointing to a certain trail! I thanked the tree and went that way, which did in fact lead me to the waterfall. In another instance I was taking a solo weekend in nature to seek guidance for my next step. At a pond where I sat for some time, there was a dead tree that looked as if it had one foot in the water, both arms outstretched, and one foot trying to reach for the nearby shore, in a sort of Tai Chi pose. The caption that popped into my mind for this humorous "tree man" was, "I'll just step out of this bog any minute now." I had to laugh at this reminder of how long I had been saying that I would make some changes in my life.

Have you ever seen the "green man"? A spirit of the forest or nature is depicted in art works of many cultures, all covered in leaves. In Native American traditions, trees are called "the standing people." The first time I noticed some very human-looking tree forms, it seemed as if their graceful mossy limbs were doing yoga poses. Recently, I observed some trees that seemed to be green men with beards, bowing rhythmically as the wind swept through them. The green men bowing to the North had big listening ears. Their bodies were marvelously fluid in their movements, shimmering and dancing, like a playing of the light in their cells.

The ocean feels very feminine to me. *La mer,* French for the ocean, is very close to *la mère,* which means mother. Sometimes she seems also like a grandmother. She teaches us to float in the feminine, open to influence, joining with the larger forces as the wave or the drop of water joins with the vast ocean. The ocean is also about change. Proteus, the god of the sea, became synonymous with changeability.

> *Sea, so gentle now*
> *I know you have bigger waves*
> *In store for me, too!*

We tend to love what is beautiful in nature, and avoid what we judge as ugly. Yet everything has its role to play; the worms eating the animal corpse are doing valuable work. Darkness has its own unique gifts; we might become more balanced if we didn't burn electric lights far into the night, but instead let the dark be dark. In the quiet darkness of not knowing, deep mystery is experienced; seeds grow. Without lights, we see the stars more clearly. Darkness is quiet, feminine, yin. It's the invisible side of the moon.

We love contrast. We would be bored in a world of only light; for depth, we need shadow. The play of light and dark fascinates us. Who doesn't love the sparkling that occurs when two contrasting substances or qualities, such as water and air, or darkness and light, interface?

> *Dark and still, the sand*
> *Yet sparkles with dancing light:*
> *Balanced yin and yang.*

On a three-day solo Vision Quest a number of years ago, I

had profound experiences of the correlation between the inner and the outer worlds. On my second night out, I dreamed of a child excitedly counting many snakes; the next day, I saw a snake several times (or perhaps there was more than one snake). In the afternoon, drowsing in the heat, my eyes closed, I had a dreamy image of a guide telling me, "The powerful spot of the circle is the center of it." As I opened my eyes, I saw the snake on a rock in the river, forming a perfect circle, head to tail! The cycle of death and rebirth is often symbolized by the *ouroborus*, the image of a snake swallowing its own tail. It is the symbol of eternity: another circle of healing. Later that day, I saw the snake gliding over the rocks just next to my sleeping bag, and felt a twinge of fear. Suddenly I decided to bring the snake's energy into myself instead of resisting it. I imagined it spinning up my spine, and felt the opening of my energy centers.

If these had been the only gifts of my quest, it would have been enough; but the best was yet to come. To my astonishment, when I returned home the true visionary fireworks were unleashed! Upon making love with my husband, I saw vivid green tropical jungles, mud, and vines; next came a golden cornucopia filled with bright yellow ears of corn and other foods, at my belly. I felt my love and appreciation for the bounty of foods. As this love became my love for the Earth, I beheld my heart as a green bud opening into the glowing pink petals of a huge flower. The love moved up into grateful songs of joy spinning from my throat, which gave rise to clear seeing through the eye of gratitude in the center of my forehead. With a burst of light out the crown, I found myself in the angelic realm. The beautiful winged ones were in throngs, so numerous, with such radiant loving white light coming from them, that I wept with joy.

CONSIDER:

- How did you experience nature as a child?
- How have you been separated from the natural world?
- Go for a walk in a park or woods. Find another being, and open up to it, listen deeply, come into its presence. Perhaps, touch it and feel its pulse, rhythm, and way of life. What can you learn?

Nature as Healer

> As long as the Earth can make a spring every year, I can.
> As long as the Earth can flower and produce nurturing
> fruit, I can, because I'm the Earth. I won't give up until
> the Earth gives up.   —Alice Walker

"When I had pneumonia," my artist friend Augusta recalls, "I would drive myself to Briones Park. I could only walk about fifteen minutes away from the road, then I'd collapse on the ground. I lay directly on the grass, or the dry creek beds. I just lay on the earth, incapable of doing anything, even visualization, to heal myself. I was just there. And then it all came in on me, and it was the most euphoric thing! I just didn't want to leave, it was like being in heaven. I was simply open, receiving. I could have died there happily. The earth healed me, and when I hike in that park now, I spend some time lying there. Sometimes that euphoria comes back. Not always."

Our true home is among the stars and trees, with crickets and frogs singing us to sleep at night, and birdsong to awaken us along with dawn light. We were meant to co-evolve with plants and creatures, not with computers and concrete. We cannot be healthy without spending time outdoors, since nature is our true source of healing energy. Healing requires an improvement in our energy flow. David Abram, author of *The Spell of the Sensuous,* believes that we need relationships with creatures other than ourselves; we can't get all our relationship needs met by humans alone. "Link your nervous system back into the ecosystem," he advises.

When I first began working with guided imagery and healing, I felt most drawn to imagery that began with a visit to a beautiful place in nature, real or imagined. In working with many clients and students, I have found this to be nearly universal. The most frequently chosen imaginary place of safety and healing is that of a secluded garden, a quiet and private place with beautiful flowers and shrubs, and birds singing in the trees. We all long for the sacred garden.

A well-known story of healing is *The Secret Garden*—a tale of two children who are healed emotionally and physically by helping restore a neglected garden. That overgrown garden is a rich metaphor for all that lies within us that has not been cared for or cultivated; it is the safe place at our deepest center, where our healing work must begin. Connection with nature is also connection with our inner nature.

One night while camping in the Grand Canyon, I awoke with an insight that felt as if it came from the depths of the Earth herself and wrote it down. In the morning, I saw that I had written: *Health is coming into proper balance with Earth energies.*

Some adults spend their vacations and weekends shopping or visiting museums. But the fresh air of the mountains and of the ocean is healing. Lie on warm sand and soak up the solar energy into all parts of your body, any parts that hurt. Or lie on leaves or pine needles and feel the support of the ground under your back. We can release unhealthy energy into the Earth, as well as receive the Earth's healing energy this way.

"We belong to the ground; it is our power and we must stay close to it; or maybe we will get lost," says Narritjin Maymuru, an Aboriginal elder.

By paying close attention to any natural entity, such as a tree, a stream, or an insect, we generate a resonance between ourselves and that healthy natural being. As we resonate, our energies become aligned; and our health is improved. If you are feeling too rushed and unable to slow down, spend time with a tree and experience its rootedness and stability. Trees are masters of tapping Earth's energy and letting it flow up through them. By attending to and appreciating these qualities, we can begin to share them. From a diverse old growth forest community, we can learn how to balance growth and death, conserve and recycle resources, and sustain ourselves through time. Luisa Teish enjoins us: "Take note of where in nature you are regenerated, and go there. Declare yourself a child of and a defender of that place. Then, live it."

When you are in the sunlight, you can see your shadow more easily. To have a shorter shadow, get close to the Earth.

Go quietly outdoors at sunset or dawn, preferably alone, and contemplate your surroundings. Notice how the creatures and plants respond to the sun's rising or setting. These times of change from day to night promote inner transformation for us. Spend time with the moon, especially if you are female or want to balance your feminine and masculine qualities.

Nature is a great storehouse of healing memories for us. Have you had a delightful experience at a beach or waterfall, or watching a sunset? Whenever we reexperience one of these, it subtly triggers the feelings of the earlier encounters and all the positive associations. For example, one of my earliest memories was of having fallen asleep in the car and being lifted in my father's gentle arms and carried into the house, aware for just a moment of the soft music of crickets and the shadows of leaves against the moonlit wall. Whenever I hear crickets now, I re-live that moment of peace and security.

Peak experiences in nature are especially healing. Once at Lake Manzanita in Mt. Lassen Park, my husband was paddling a little inflatable raft and I swam up to it and pulled myself in. The contrast between the cool, refreshing water and the hot sun on my skin, with the snow-capped mountain above and blue sky all around me, sent me into an extraordinarily blissful state. A duck with five ducklings swam alongside the raft and I was ecstatic. Now, the sight of ducklings evokes very warm and happy feelings for me.

Of course, we can reexperience these feelings through our imagination as well, without a stimulus to elicit them. One of my favorite memories is of swimming up behind a waterfall on the island of Kauai and embracing the wet green moss on the ancient black volcanic rock. It felt as if I had come home to a deep place of oneness with Mother Earth.

Regular visits to places of natural beauty are essential for me. to "charge up my green batteries." Feasting my eyes on the myriad shades of green in an area with trees and plants rejuvenates me. Trees breathing, moving, rooting, evaporating, condensing, moistening, growing, standing, sheltering, pointing, teaching.

Try walking barefooted, in places where it is safe to do so. Thich Nhat Hanh advises, "Walk as if your feet were giving love-pats to Mother Earth." These bodies were designed to receive sensory input from the Earth through our feet. How many of our foot, leg, and knee problems result from not feeling the surface we walk on? Walking barefoot on sand gives an excellent workout to legs and feet, and may confer some of the benefits experienced in a session of reflexology, acupressure or a foot massage. Some believe that the sensations received through the feet can fine-tune our entire nervous system as well. Studies show that the surface we walk upon even influences the way we breathe. High, shallow chest breathing occurs more frequently when we walk on pavement than when we walk on grass or earth. This same breath pattern is associated with "fight or flight," a state of nervous arousal that is part of the body's stress response. Experiment with taking your shoes off. Do you notice that you step more lightly, carefully, and slowly? Bare feet are alive feet that connect us to the Earth. We feel more grounded, without having to experience heaviness. By standing barefoot on the Earth and giving our attention to the sensations we feel, we receive energy directly through the soles of our feet.

Indigenous peoples the world over recognize the need for periodic healing of the relationships between humans and nature. Illnesses, droughts, and bad luck in hunting have been thought to be caused by spirits. Shamans are those who serve as intermediaries, and help to restore the balance and harmony between humans and the spirits that dwell in nature. Their ability to heal people arises as a byproduct of their connectedness with both worlds. Indigenous peoples live in much closer contact and relationship with nature than us "civilized" folk. And yet, they have institutionalized rituals and shamans to tend the boundary between humans and nature. How much more do WE need shamans! Now some anthropologists, ecopsychologists, and healers are studying and engaging in shamanic practices. Modern shamans may assist people in finding a wise "power animal" through shamanic journeying to the beat of a drum; or, they may lead people on Vision Quests in secluded natural places in order to discover their life purpose.

Our society as a whole, however, still regards such practices as quaint superstition, completely without value except to "primitive," uneducated folk.

A component of shamanism is the understanding that all beings are deeply interconnected at the spirit level. When we touch or embrace a tree, we are in communion. I have noticed how my thoughts and mood change as I spend time in close contact with a redwood, pine or cedar tree. Have you ever smelled the bark of a Jeffrey pine? It is an indescribable mixture of vanilla, cinnamon, and nuts. David Abram suggests that when we walk through the woods, we are not only seeing, hearing, touching, and smelling, but also *being* seen, heard, touched, smelled. The wind and trees, he says, speak when a breeze moves through their branches, just as we speak when air passes through our vocal cords. We can commune and connect by singing, humming, talking, or even whistling to the creatures and plants. Many people speak to their house plants, as well as to their animal pets. How about talking to trees and animals encountered on a walk in nature?

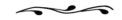

FOREST GRACE
Huckleberry, you touch my hair
With a lover's gentle care.
Ferns, you grow so near the path
And softly contact all who pass.
Bird sings two notes; I whistle back two.
Now you sing three; will I follow you?
Wordless communion of touch and sound:
I once was lost, but now am found.

We would probably all agree that love is the greatest healer. Yet what a challenge it often is to love ourselves, our friends, or our neighbors; perhaps it is most difficult of all to love certain members of our family! What if loving ourselves and other humans were the two most difficult kinds of love? Wouldn't it be helpful to practice loving in some easier ways, too?

Dogs and cats are loving and adorable, and that mutual love is healing. Pets can help lower their owners' blood pressure and decrease heart attacks. Nursing homes that brought in plants and animals reported a 40 percent decrease in death rates, as well as a major reduction in patients' loneliness and depression. Hospital and nursing home patients receive great benefits from even occasional visits with animals. In the Prison Pet Partnership Program, service dogs are raised and trained by women inmates. The women leave as fully qualified pet technicians, and since 1988 none of them have been repeat offenders. Many of the women are mothers, and prison officials have noted that their parenting skills improve as a result of their interactions with the dogs. Perhaps it becomes easier to love humans when we are also in a loving connection with some of the other beings with whom we share this planet.

Planting a garden and spending time there is beneficial to both body and soul. A good garden is a gift from the Earth. It helps us to cultivate ourselves, which was Voltaire's great advice. Whatever we do outwardly can be a metaphor for inner experience as well. As Rachel Naomi Remen eloquently says, in her book *Kitchen Table Wisdom*, "The way we tend the life force in a plant may be the way we tend our own life force."

Eating food we grow ourselves puts us in touch with the source of the food; we have a relationship with it instead of eating mindlessly. The fresher the food when we eat it, the more of Earth's healing and nourishing energy is still within it. Foods were not intended to be harvested thousands of miles away and shipped and refrigerated for weeks before consumption, nor were they meant to be processed through machines, doused with chemicals, and packaged in plastic. The closer we are to eating naturally (organic vegetables, fruits, whole grains), the easier it is to acknowledge the Source. The more we appreciate our food, the more it nurtures us. Whenever you feel deprived or lacking, go study the abundance of a blackberry bush, an apple tree, or an evergreen.

As our environment degrades, some of us are becoming more sensitive: to the chemicals in the air and the water, to the burning rays of the sun due to loss of protective ozone. This increase in sensitivity gives us another opportunity to wake up. My hope is that we will become more and more motivated to take action to reverse the environmental degradation.

Do something, even insignificant, to give back to the Earth. Service to the planet is service to humanity. An important role for the elders of our time is to teach children reverence for nature and protection of the Earth. Even picking up a single piece of trash from a natural place is a loving act. As soon as I decide to pick up some litter, a plastic bag in which to collect it will usually appear. Clean up the places in nature where you want to spend time. Help bring back the natural beauty of some part of the neighborhood where you live, or a park, a beach, or a creek. It's amazing how good I feel when I remove a bunch of plastic trash from a beach; I can feel a huge "thank you" from the ocean. Ken Carey, author of *Return of the Bird Tribes*, says that when we succeed in cleaning up our mental toxins, it will become a simple matter to clean up the environmental ones. I like to think that it works both ways.

I pledge allegiance to the Earth:
I will honor this body given me by birth.
The body is my connection with the Mother;
If I pollute one, then I pollute the other.
The unity of body and mind
Brings peace and wisdom to humankind.

Once I had a dream in which a group of furry brown monsters had wrought terrible environmental degradation. They
were climbing a snowy hill that was bare of trees. Perhaps these
monsters represented us humans, who have done so much
despoiling of the earth and cutting of forests. Suddenly their
furry coats split open, and out popped the robust branches of
evergreen trees! A great transformation had occurred. The
trees stood on the hill in all their glory, and the mountain was
forested again.

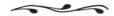

CONSIDER: How do you tend your own life force?
     What are your ideal conditions for growth?

The Winged Ones

Did you think this section was going to be about birds? No,
it's about winged insects. They fascinate me, and they gift us
humans with visits more than most other wild creatures do. I
like to think of winged ones as a special class of beings that
includes butterflies, dragonflies, all sorts of flies, bees, mosquitoes, and flying beetles, as well as bats, birds, and angels.
     In our culture insects are almost universally hated, except for
butterflies, ladybugs, and a few others that are pretty to look at.

People think nothing of killing insects, considering them a nuisance. I never realized quite how deeply this hatred is felt until, in a workshop on edible wild plants, I discovered that two of my classmates were in business as exterminators! They thought of themselves as lovers of nature, while making an exception for insects.

Caroline Myss, a renowned intuitive with a strong Catholic background, advises us to look for the most powerful forces in the smallest and humblest packages, citing the example of Jesus's birth in the manger. Insects are some of the tiniest creatures with whom we share this planet.

Joanne Lauck, in *The Voice of the Infinite in the Small: Revisioning the Human-Insect Connection*, points out that we have projected a lot of our shadow upon insects. If we can heal the human-insect relationship, it will be a giant step toward re-owning our collective shadow. We need to set boundaries with insects, asking them to respect our living spaces or our vegetable gardens, but we can do so with respect, and even with a blessing. Our efforts to eradicate insects with pesticides are not only endangering our health and that of many other creatures, but also destroying a part of our inner selves. In Navajo mythology, according to Lauck, Big Fly is revered as a mediator between people and their gods, and frequently lights near the ear of a person who needs instruction. We depend on bees and butterflies to pollinate our crops; other insects aerate the soil, recycle our wastes, and serve as food for countless species.

I have experienced assistance from a fly coming very near my face to warn me to pay attention to what was right in front of me. I had nearly walked into some poison oak! Once, while I was debating between two courses of action, I was sure that a fly sang happily into my ear, "Whatever serves the highest purpose."

In his classic, *Kinship with All Life,* J. Allen Boone relates the story of an affectionate and respectful relationship with a housefly, "Freddie," who enjoyed playing games and having his wings stroked, as well as communicating in the silent language of the heart. Freddie would not come near one visitor who held insects in contempt, even when the man professed respect and admiration; the little fly saw through him.

A large part of what heals me in nature is the sense of communion. This goes beyond the communication of teachings and guidance, as wonderful as that is. When I am in a self-judging mood, mosquitoes seem to come and bite me more, as if mirroring my attacks. But once in awhile, when a mosquito lands on my arm, I remember what the Dalai Lama said: "When the first mosquito comes, I say 'Help yourself.'" On a couple of occasions when I've done that, an extraordinary thing happened: the mosquito stayed for many minutes, and I had a wonderful sense of sharing a bit of my abundance (after all, a lot less than the local medical lab or blood bank takes). I even sent a pulsation of love from my heart, through the bloodstream to the mosquito. When my visitor finally left, there was no sting, no itch, no swelling anywhere.

> *Hello, mosquito.*
> *I don't need acupuncture*
> *Since you befriend me.*

Bird Talk

But ask now the beasts, and they shall teach thee;
And the fowls of the air, and they shall teach thee.

—Job 12:7

"Say thank you!" prompted the bird. I looked up, startled. It was unmistakable: the very same inflection that my mother had used with us ungrateful children when we had been given a gift. Since the bird persisted in singing those three notes, I decided to do as I was told. As soon as I made the decision to be grateful, my bad mood lifted. After all, it was a beautiful, sunny, warm day; I was about to embark on a three-day solo Vision Quest, which I had been anticipating for many weeks. Certain things were not happening according to my expectations, but that just meant it was time to let go of those expectations.

Birds often live near where people are; it seems to me that they know and use our inflections sometimes. In *The Spell of the Sensuous*, David Abram writes about a tribe of Alaskan Indians, the Koyukon, who have many words in their language taken from bird calls. "Once, some years ago, people heard a horned owl clearly intone the Koyukon words 'Black bears will cry.' For the next two seasons, the wild berry crops failed and many bears found it hard to survive." In another account of the Koyukon, a grey jay spoke "in an uncommonly human voice" during a rainstorm: 'My brother . . . my brother, what is going to happen?'. . . Afterward the rain poured down for nine days, flooding bears from their dens and creating general havoc. And then people knew what the bird had meant."

Alex, an African gray parrot trained by Dr. Irene Pepperberg, learned to answer the questions, "What color?" and "What shape?" with over 80 percent accuracy. He could also answer "How many?" correctly 95 percent of the time, according to Donald Griffin, author of *Animal Minds*.

I am keenly aware of birds as my allies when they seem to dialogue with thoughts I am having. Here are some excerpts.

Thought: I'll take time off.
Bird: *To do your sweet work.*

Thought: I judge myself as unproductive.
Bird: *A pity.*

Thought: I'm not likely to be a very good teacher ...
Bird: *Yet!*

Thought: Instead of negativity, I could try ...
Bird: *Music, prayer! Believe in music prayer!*

Thought: I'll learn some Earth prayers.
Bird: *Sweet!*

Thought: I might take a day in nature, once a month.
Bird: *Just try it once!*

Thought: To say yes when I mean no is dishonest to myself.
Bird: *Isn't polite!*

Thought: I'll learn to open my heart in nature.
Bird: *True! Pure!*

Thought: I'll make relationship more important than the material things.
Bird: *It is!*

Thought: I want to see a change in people's attitudes.
Bird: *Be it! Be it! Be it!*

A Swainson's thrush, with upward-spiraling melodic triplets, instructed me thus:

> *Linear, linear thinking*
> *Doesn't go anywhere.*
> *Upward thinking does. Try spiral logic.*
> *We're bringing you peace, peace, peace!*

At various times, birds have enjoined me to wake up, slow down, get closer to the ground, listen, forgive, and even to pick up paper off a beach. I've received several lectures about living a healthier lifestyle, getting more exercise and purifying my diet. Many times when I've had sad thoughts, I've heard a bird singing a mournful, downward moving scale. Often, if I'm having an important insight, they seem to say, *Yes! Yes!* so that I won't discount the idea as insignificant. One day, just as it occurred to me that a certain group I belonged to needed to do some brainstorming, a group of birds began making excited sounds like several people tossing out ideas all at once.

Another time, as I contemplated working on this book, I became aware of a steady bird sound that seemed to go on for nearly an hour. It reminded me of something, but I couldn't place it. Finally, I recognized that it was very close to the sound of fingers typing on a keyboard. Am I projecting all this meaning onto the birds' sounds? Probably! But then, according to many metaphysical teachings, we are the ones who assign meaning to everything that occurs in our lives.

> *Bird gives a sermon*
> *To me, from its lofty perch;*
> *Or a serenade?*

One day in Marble Mountain Wilderness, I took a solo hike

and sat down to rest and meditate. Opening my eyes, I found myself surrounded by hummingbirds, tiny harbingers of joy. They flew all around me, chirping and whirring, some very close, darting in a wild dance. One came near me, drinking from a bright orange-red Indian paintbrush flower. "Go for the beauty and sweetness," it seemed to admonish me, and buzzed me loudly from behind with its whirring wings, as if to show it meant business!

One of Many Bright Blades Emerging Triumphant Through the Concrete

There are many and there will be many more to follow, spreading greenness, spreading Green news. Life is determined to emerge past all the manmade layers placed on the skin of Mother Earth. There is no stopping the exuberant force of spring, there is no stopping an idea whose time has come. There is nothing that cannot be overcome by the power of tiny fragile beings in large numbers. Greenness is manifold. There is grass over all the earth, in fields and prairies, under summer sun and autumn rain; it will green the world, we will green this world once again. No one knows where the mysterious life force will sprout forth, through what rubble of manmade mindless malevolence. What is this urge for growth? It is the same as a thunderhead pregnant with rain, ready to burst; the same as a throat full of music aching to be sung. The movement to reclaim the Earth is growing, spreading, sprouting up at kitchen tables, in schoolrooms, in churches, in corporations, irrepressible!

Invoking Sacred Space

*Where ritual is absent, the young ones are restless or
violent, there are no real elders, and the grown-ups are
bewildered. The future is dim.* —Malidoma Somé

Rituals are formulas by which harmony is restored.
—Terry Tempest-Williams

Malidoma Somé, a West African healer from a small tribal village who came to the United States and obtained two doctorates, left his position at Brandeis at the urging of his village elders in order to devote his life to teaching Westerners about ritual. He believes that the lack of ritual in the modern Western world is responsible for the great social problems we face. "In the absence of ritual," he writes, "the soul runs out of its real nourishment."

How did our society become so illiterate in the ways of ritual? The Catholic Church tortured and burned "witches," primarily women who were herbalists, or used spells or rituals to invoke spiritual forces. We were seduced by science and rationalism, taught to scoff at ritual as "unscientific mumbo-jumbo" practiced by "uncivilized" people. Important rituals such as baptisms, weddings, and funerals were institutionalized, placed in the hands of priests and ministers, funeral directors and doctors. These ceremonies did not allow for participation or spontaneity; rarely did they evoke a true sense of the sacred. Most of our modern rituals have been removed from nature and the elements.

Today, there is a resurgence of interest in rituals, as well as in the indigenous peoples who have kept them alive. As ancient as humankind, rituals were practiced by all traditional cultures. The essence of ritual is to call upon the invisible world of spirit for assistance or guidance with the things we know we can't manage by ourselves. In *Making the Gods Work for You*, Caroline Casey refers to ritual as "the language of the gods," which we must learn to use if we wish to have their help. Christina Baldwin, author of *Calling the Circle*, reminds us that "ritual in the circle is the way we invite collective wisdom and acknowledge spiritual center." Her book describes how council circles can help resolve conflicts and heal entire communities.

By creating the physical embodiment of an abstract concept, ritual can dramatize and make the concept real for the participants; thus it provides a wonderful means of teaching values to the young. We can plant a seed in the ground to represent what we wish to nurture in ourselves, or light a candle to symbolize our wish for illumination. Since rituals often include objects, actions, singing, and/or dancing, they involve many parts of us other than our logical, problem-solving left brains. They communicate on a deeper, more universal level.

Ritual is a metaphoric language which can tap into the universal archetypes of the human unconscious, our ancestral heritage. By performing ceremonies which have been done for centuries, we invite ancient collective wisdom. Through ritual, we increase balance and connection within ourselves, with the natural world, and with the spirit realm. In shamanic traditions, rituals are used for calling upon the spirit world for assistance in healing the sick.

In their book *The Art of Ritual*, Sydney Metrick and Renee

Beck describe ritual as a marker of life's significant events and transitions, a buffer for change, and a bridge between the inner and outer worlds. They believe that planning and participating in ritual gives us a sense of creative power, helping us to cope with life's inevitable endings and losses, and to view them from a broader perspective. Ritual can help us overcome our resistance to change, and provide containment for strong emotions.

Matthew Fox, author of *Original Blessing*, is a former Dominican priest ousted by the Pope for his earth-centered spiritual teachings. He founded the University of Creation Spirituality and a ritual center in downtown Oakland, California, where his group regularly holds ecumenical "techno-cosmic masses." At these events there are invocations, altars, dancing to live music, and rap performances, while multiple images are projected kaleidoscopically upon all the walls. There is grieving, celebration, and communion. When a group of doctors took part in a techno-cosmic mass in celebration of the human body, several of them told Fox that the ritual had restored their reverence for the mystery and beauty of the body and expressed the wish that they had experienced this sense of awe as part of their medical training. Fox believes that ritual must be meaningful to youth, and sees it as "an indispensable element for authentic community because in it we come together to name and celebrate, to lament, grieve, and let go and to create and recreate our common task: the Great Work of the Universe."

Rituals can be co-created by large or small groups, or done on one's own. They can be elaborate or simple; they can follow a tradition or be created on the spot. In order to invoke the assistance of the spirit world, people have followed certain practices for thousands of years: creating altars and sacred circles, cleansing themselves, honoring and calling upon spirit helpers, and working with the elements of fire, air, water, and earth.

Energy may be centered by physically forming a circle of people or of stones, and perhaps by breathing together or sounding a bell. To breathe together is literally to "conspire." Drumming, singing or chanting, and dancing raise the spiritual energy, which is then directed into symbolic actions. Finally the energy is grounded and integrated; this may occur by passing a talking stick so that those present may share how they will internalize the ritual. Touching the Earth is also grounding.

To invoke sacred space is to invite ourselves into a circle that exists outside of everyday space and time, where even ordinary actions take on special meaning.

> *The dramatic action that we need to create a way of life on Earth that really works will be taken not through personal, social or political action, but through spiritual action.*   —Brooke Medicine Eagle

Humble Beginnings

First, and possibly most important, is the attitude and practice of humility. What keeps us humble truly lifts us up. Humility means being close to the humus, the soil; being willing to learn from the Earth, including her insects; to listen more than we speak. It is knowing that the smallest, most easily overlooked can be the most powerful teacher. Humility is being small in appearance and large of heart.

We acknowledge our weakness and admit that we don't know how to bring about the results we want, without assistance from Spirit. We give all credit for any accomplishments to Spirit.

Performing a symbolic cleansing or purification helps us set aside our small-minded selves, occupied with petty concerns.

This is often done by burning sage or cedar, and wafting the smoke over each participant to clear their energy fields. Or, a few drops of water may be sprinkled on each person's head.

One of my favorite rituals is to bow to Mother Earth, touching my forehead to the ground, while acknowledging all of Earth's gifts, and asking for Earth wisdom. Have you thought of bowing to your mother, or your children? How about all of Earth's children? Once I bowed to a horse, struck with its beauty, and received several light kisses on top of my head!

Realizing how insignificant I am enlivens my sense of humor. Part of humility is remembering that I don't know what anything is for, that I don't see the master plan. I don't need to understand exactly what the gift is, or when it's going to arrive.

Once we have loosened the grip of the judgmental mind and opened up through symbolic cleansing and humility, we begin to create space for the sacred to unfold. Being quiet in nature helps to still the overly dominant language-making part of our minds. As we slow down and begin to listen, we open the door to the more-than-human world. At those moments we become aware that everything has meaning.

Altared States

Create an altar for your ritual. It can have on it a symbol of each element: fire, air, earth, and water. An altar can portray the balance of these elements, as you might wish them to be balanced in nature and in yourself.

A candle can represent fire, which is related to inspiration. Air is an element linked with mental clarity; it is often symbolized by a bird feather. The earth can be represented by a stone or crystal, a flower, a piece of fruit or other food. The earth element signifies completion, manifestation, and grounding. And water, linked with emotion and flow, can be placed in a vessel or symbolized by a seashell. Metrick and Beck link the four elements with the four directions, placing fire in the South, air in the East, earth in the North, and water in the West.

A special symbol may be placed on the altar to represent the particular issue with which you are working. For example, a broken stick might represent a broken relationship that needs healing; a chambered nautilus shell could signify growth into a new phase of life. Or you could draw a picture.

Creating a simple altar in nature can be a highly symbolic act. As you place each natural treasure on your altar, you may create a design of bird feathers, colorful stones, pine cones, and the like. Every object has meaning. Some indigenous peoples believe that stones are our wise elders, carrying the memory of the earth.

To create beauty by arranging things artistically is a natural act that gives us joy. Contemplate what each object means to you and why you gathered it. When you get very close to the pebbles on a beach, you can see that each one has a story. This one is from Japan: a perfect Zen stone, black and square with simple clean white lines. Here is a luminous jade teardrop from China. Now I see an African mask of brown and topaz.

When your ritual or meditation is finished, return each item to its former place with thanks.

Rituals of Honoring

> *Rituals, especially the rituals of the sacred circle—the*
> *hoop of life which contains all things—remind us that we*
> *all spring from the center, the source, the All-That-Is; that*
> *the aliveness of the Great Spirit lives in each of us; and*
> *that we all have an equal place in things. In remembering,*
> *we can again become members of the Great Family. The*
> *four-legged, wingeds, the rock people and green growing*
> *ones are inviting us now to awaken and step again with*
> *love fully into that great circle. Let us find good relation-*
> *ship with all things in a daily ritual—be it inner, outer,*
> *silent, or sung—for all our relatives.*
>
> —Brooke Medicine Eagle

An essential aspect of ritual is honoring the place we are in. Honoring the four directions is a tradition practiced by Native Americans and many others. It is done for all major cere-monies, such as the solstices and equinoxes, as part of the lay-ing of a Medicine Wheel, and for sweat lodges and vision quests. One reason I love this ritual is that my own sense of direction was so poor that I could get lost in a parking lot— another reason why I hate shopping malls. Although I am gradually recovering, I carry a compass with me to find north. Honoring the directions helps us to feel centered in the sacred circle, and to attune ourselves to everything around us. Facing each direction, observe whatever is there, naming it and thanking it, and asking it to share its blessings.

In Sun Bear's Medicine Wheel tradition, certain animals are the "spirit keepers" for the four directions.

North is the direction of wisdom of the white-haired elders, purity, presence, leadership, winter, and the White Buffalo.

Facing north, I may see a tall tree, and acknowledge the northerly qualities of the tree. Or I may behold a white cloud or feel a cool breeze coming from the north.

East carries the awakening energies of sunrise, spring, and new beginnings; its gift is the far-seeing vision of the Eagle. The color is yellow or gold. Inspiration and illumination, the opening of the third eye, and enlightenment are associated with this direction. Often I notice yellow flowers as I face east.

South holds the energies of childlike trust and innocence, summer, the heart's healing path, and the playful trickster Coyote who makes us laugh at ourselves. If, while facing south, I see water flowing in that direction, I might notice the trustful ability of water to let go and flow freely, and its playfulness as it bubbles happily over the rocks. Red is a color often associated with south; when red birds fly toward me from the south, they may be messengers from that direction.

West is the direction of the setting sun, darkness, ocean, autumn, and the introspective insight of the Bear. In facing the west, we face the shadow, and let go of attachments (a kind word that includes addictions). That, to me, can be scary stuff! The setting sun reminds us that great beauty comes in letting go, and loveliness comes out of loss.

Laying a stone for each of the four directions establishes a sacred circle. In some traditions, there are six directions, so that Mother Earth and Father Sky are always included. To honor Mother Earth I touch my forehead to the ground, asking Earth to share her wisdom and insight with me and thanking her for all her gifts. While standing or sitting, I imagine my roots going down from the base of my spine to ground me firmly in the Earth, and to nourish me with her energy. Looking up, I thank and honor Father Sky/Father Sun for light and beauty and warmth, and helping all things grow.

The elements of water, air, earth, and fire are sacred. If a stream, lake, or ocean is near, I usually take a few drops and sprinkle them on my head, acknowledging the purifying qualities of water. Or I may take some from my water bottle to drink and sprinkle it. If it is a very dry place, I might share some of my water with the plants or trees there. To honor the air, conscious breathing with gratitude for its gift of life is the best way I know. When a group takes a few breaths together, they join on a deep level. Observe from which direction a breeze or wind is blowing, and understand it as a messenger from that direction. Fire can be honored through Father Sun, or lighting a candle. Earth, the rich humus that supports life, is so often dishonored (as in "dirty hands"). Holding some earth in my hand, I appreciate and thank it. Offering a pinch of cornmeal is another way to honor Earth by giving something back.

Seeing all in nature as our relatives was a practice of St. Francis of Assisi, who referred to "Sister Moon" and "Brother Bird." It is also a practice in most Native American traditions, emphasizing our kinship with "Grandmother Spider" and "Father Sun." A very brief but complete prayer is simply: "All my relations" (Ho mitakuye oyasin, in Lakota).

After thus invoking sacred space, we are supported by all the spirits of the land for help in what we wish to accomplish. The next step is to clarify and state intention. What problem or issue are we facing, and what outcome or understanding would we like?

Seasonal Rituals

Some of the most important rituals for the human family are those that honor the Earth's movement through the circle of seasons: the equinoxes and solstices. Since before recorded history, our ancestors have done rituals to celebrate the coming of each new season; and when we take part in these observances, we tap into the powerful energy field echoing to us across the generations. Many of our Christian and Jewish holidays are synchronous with these sacred times. This may be seen as a strategic move on the part of the newer religions to take over and replace the old pagan traditions, or it may be viewed as an aspect of universality in all faiths.

Imagine a rusty old wheel that creaks when set into motion, representing the ways in which we get out of touch with the natural cycles. Seasonal rituals are like oiling and moving the wheel, to bring us back into harmony with the energy of nature, so that our lives become less effortful, more balanced with the natural flow. We celebrate the changes we observe in the earth and sun, and also note the changes taking place within ourselves. It is believed that the times of seasonal transition provide moments when the veil between the apparent physical world and the invisible spirit world is thinner and more permeable. Thus the spirits are more able to hear us and to aid us.

The seasons of the year are linked with the four directions, and also are strongly associated with the stages of human life: spring (east, infancy, new beginnings), summer (south, childhood/adolescence, rapid growth), fall (west, middle age, letting go), and winter (north, old age, inwardness). As we progress through the wheel of the seasons, we have the opportunity to try out or revisit each of these life stages, always with a new perspective.

Being present and aware of where we stand in the turning of the year can inform our rituals. It's wonderful to do rituals of gathering, harvesting, completion, and letting go during the autumn, and rituals of planting new seeds and beginning new endeavors in the spring. If I am trying to start new things in the fall, I need to be prepared for resistance and difficulty, because I have not aligned myself with the rhythms and cycles of nature.

The equinoxes, times when the night and day are of equal length, are reminders to bring ourselves back into balance; balance of light and dark, male and female, earth and sky. Co-creating group rituals is a splendid way to strengthen the bonds of community.

For more ideas about seasonal rituals, see *The Ceremonial Circle* by Sedonia Cahill, *The Medicine Wheel* and other books by Sun Bear, and *The Spiral Dance* by Starhawk.

Rituals with Personal Meaning

> *Ritual is the act of sanctifying action—even ordinary*
> *action—so that it has meaning: I can light a candle*
> *because I need the light or because the candle represents*
> *the light I need.*   —Christina Baldwin

My older sister and I had been adversaries since childhood. Less than two years younger, I beat her at most games and got my driver's license before she did. My friends and I would conspire to make her life miserable. As adults, we were not close geographically or emotionally.

In June 1995, I invited her to go camping with me in Yosemite, intending to heal our relationship in a place we had loved visiting as children. The first day brought out the worst in both of us. Having overlooked the fact that my sister had little experience with camping, I was taken aback by her anxiety and helplessness. In my harshly judgmental eyes, my sister seemed terribly neurotic and needy. Malevolently, I harbored fantasies of throwing myself into one of the raging waterfalls. "A murder-suicide in reverse!" I thought, darkly. "If I killed myself, everyone would blame her for driving me to such desperation. That would do her in completely."

Then, on the summer solstice, we took a hike up the so-called "Mist" trail, past Vernal Falls. It had been a wet winter, and the torrential waterfall drenched everyone on the trail! At the top, having received a thorough cleansing from the powerful white cascade of pure snowmelt, people were in high spirits. Laughing and shivering, hikers squeezed water out of their garments and spread them on rocks to dry in the bright sun. There was a sense of community among total strangers from all over the globe, united by our common experience. Although she had feared slipping and tumbling into the falls, my sister felt a thrill of accomplishment for surviving the intense ascent. I felt washed clean of my toxic thoughts by the waterfall.

On the return loop, I couldn't help staring at a T-shirt which proclaimed: LIFE IS SHORT PRAY HARD! (Read the Book). Its owner was a friendly fellow who was hiking with his wife. He became my spiritual adviser, while his wife engaged my sister in friendly conversation, walking behind us. As I shared my troubled thoughts with him, he spoke to me of how all families experience conflict. "We needn't be perfect," he consoled me. "Just ask your sister's forgiveness, and be willing to accept it." He counseled me to slow down and listen more to her feelings. I felt as if an angel had been placed in my path. "My wife and I like to help people," he said simply.

After this magical solstice experience, I felt inspired to do a ritual with my sister for putting our past behind us. We picked up some sticks and waged a mock battle with them to represent our past conflicts, then stood on a bridge over a river and dropped them on the upstream side. Moving to watch the sticks float downstream, we said, "That's all water under the bridge." Then we found a twig with two leaves on it, to represent the new and living relationship, and "planted" it under the parent tree. We have a picture of the two of us holding our twig; and we often sign our letters with a sketch of the twig with its two leaves. The ritual helped us to open up to each other more about some previously unshared things in our personal lives, and we committed to a monthly phone call to stay more in touch. Our relationship still has many problems, but we feel much more connected.

For personal rituals, I like to begin by finding the place that attracts or calls to me. If possible, I choose a place where I am not able to see human traces in any direction, and I bring a minimum of human-made items with me. To avoid the ubiquitous sounds of planes, cars, and machines, I often go to a place with natural sounds of its own, such as a running stream or waterfall. Sometimes, however, human-made elements can be part of the sacred space; for example, a bridge over a river may have a symbolic meaning in my life.

Opening up all my senses in nature helps me move from a narrow, ego focus to a broader awareness. An easy way to do this is to shift into "wide-angle vision": a softer gaze that allows me to see a large panorama. Or, by closing my eyes, I invite my other senses to open. It's amazing how much more I hear and feel with my eyes closed, such as the distant humming of insects, or the subtle sensations of warmth and shade on different parts of my body.

According to Brooke Medicine Eagle, healing through ritual action is enhanced when we create an intense emotional charge. For example, for a person needing to take the leap out of her comfort zone in order to enter a new career, a ritual action might be jumping off a ledge that is high enough to be a bit scary and exhilarating.

For making a transition in my life, one of my favorite rituals is to stand on one side of a river and consider where I am now and where I want to be. A river that is challenging to maneuver, requiring careful choices of stepping stones, works well. As I cross the river I affirm who I am becoming. Upon reaching the other side, I declare that I have now accomplished the steps and arrived at my goal. This is great to do aloud, with another person as a witness.

The new moon is said to be the most auspicious time for planting seeds; it is thus a favorable time for making plans or initiating a new activity. The full moon is a time for celebrating harvest and completion, expressing gratitude for what has been reaped.

Sunset, the time of transition from daylight to darkness, is a powerful time for rituals and prayers for release. According to Angeles Arrien, the west is the direction associated with letting go in many indigenous traditions. Some physical problems that are linked with difficulty in letting go might be: back pain (carrying too many burdens), constipation, and jaw pain.

There are many ways to do rituals of letting go and moving on. A time-honored way to let go is to write down what you wish to release on a piece of paper and then ceremonially burn it in a fire. This is especially powerful when done with others. Winter solstice or New Year's Eve are traditional occasions for this ceremony. Additionally, one may write down and offer to the flames a positive intention, thus sending it up to Spirit with the smoke of the fire. Or, the new intention may be planted with prayers in the ground, or wrapped with yarn around a "prayer arrow" and launched into moving water. We can literally sweat out our impurities and shortcomings in the prayerful atmosphere of a sweat lodge.

Try loading a backpack with stones until it feels heavy but not overwhelming. Let each stone represent a burden you want to release. Carry the pack for awhile, feeling its weight and your discomfort. Release one stone at a time, while declaring what you would like to let go of. Enjoy the lightening of your pack. How many stones are you willing to unload? Contemplate: "What, in me, makes it difficult to release these burdens?" You may decide to keep less than half of your stones. Name the ones you are keeping. Remember to thank the stones for their participation in your ritual of release, and return them to where you found them.

If letting go feels too difficult, a ritual can help to redefine it as fun and easy. For example, you might drop flower petals onto the ground one by one, while stating silently or aloud that letting go is as easy as dropping petals, as inconsequential, as lovely. Try writing, sculpting, or sketching what you wish to release in moist sand at a beach, and letting the waves erase it. Or go to a playground where there is a sandbox and some children; make your sculpture or structure there, and invite a child to destroy it for you. No child has ever refused me this favor! Letting go might be as much of a relief as releasing urine from an over-full bladder. Each time you urinate, or whenever you remember, silently remind yourself what you are letting go of.

Do you feel difficulty in completing a task or accomplishing things? You might choose a small peak you know you can climb in an hour or so. In Point Reyes, it takes me less than an hour and a half to go from the parking lot to the top of Mt. Wittenberg at a comfortable pace. All the way up, remind yourself of whatever goal you have. Notice if the desire to quit arises, and keep going anyway, remembering that this accomplishment will have ripples of resonance into many parts of your life. Once at the top, congratulate yourself for your success.

If a group is suffering from poor communication or some other internal division, a lovely way to promote healing is to ask everyone to take hands in a circle and breathe together. With each breath, imagine filling up with light, until the individual lights begin to blend and fill the room with radiant energy and well-being.

When going through a great loss, ritual can help us experience our grief, find meaning, and gain spiritual perspective. Since my mother, Louisa, was never religious and tended to avoid churches, the family decided to plan her memorial service. Leafing through a hastily-purchased book, I found a simple ceremony that appealed to me. We purchased a large box of votive candles, and one of my mother's friends brought a tall, special candle which was lit and placed in front of an enlarged photograph of Louisa. Each person present was invited to light a votive using the flame of "Louisa's candle" and say a few words about how she had brought light into their lives. Despite the intense heat of the August afternoon, one person after the other came forward to light a candle and share a reminiscence or an appreciation, until nearly everyone present had done so. There was not a dry eye to be seen. My brother, sister and I learned so much about what our mother had meant to her friends, colleagues, and clients through that simple ritual.

For more ideas on healing and ritual, listen to Brooke Medicine Eagle's audiotape, *Healing through Ritual Action.*

Opening the Circle

Before leaving your sacred circle, take a moment to thank the four directions by turning in a counterclockwise fashion to acknowledge each. This opens the circle and shares the blessings with all. It often seems to me that I reap the most profound teachings from each direction at that moment.

Beyond Materialism

*As you simplify your life, the laws of the universe will be
simpler.* —Henry David Thoreau

*If you let go of trying to get more of what you don't really
need, it frees up unbelievable amounts of energy to make
a difference with what you already have.* —Lynne Twist

By high school graduation, our kids have watched an
estimated 360,000 commercials, and will have spent
more time watching ads than in the classroom. They
are being indoctrinated in the consumer religion: fulfillment
through buying. Ninety-three percent of teenage girls in America state that their favorite activity is shopping at the mall. By
the time they are seven years old, many girls have already
learned to hate their own bodies. The average mother shops
six hours a week, and plays with her children less than one
hour a week. We Americans consume far more than our share
of the planet's resources. With four percent of the world's pop-
ulation, we consume twenty times as much as people in third-
world nations, and four times as much as people in other
industrialized nations. To provide all six billion people on this
planet with the lifestyle of the average North American would
require at least three additional Earths!

Yet, with our ever-increasing material living standard, we are not generally happier. Advertising must cultivate dissatisfaction, greed, and loneliness to motivate us to consume more. Overconsumption not only impoverishes others whose land, labor, and resources subsidize our affordable products. It also creates pollution, waste, and environmental degradation worldwide, and robs resources from our own grandchildren.

The Australian Aborigines say, "To wound the earth is to wound yourself, and if others wound the earth, they are wounding you." And as David Abram expressed it in *The Spell of the Sensuous:* "The whole Earth is straining to remind us that the planet is our own flesh, the rivers our own blood."

At some point, Mother Earth will slap us out of our consumer daze, our computer craze, and our commuter haze. Or, we can voluntarily choose a more sustainable lifestyle, realizing that our greatest resources are the inner ones.

When the reward of work is intrinsic rather than extrinsic, we are healthier emotionally. The satisfaction of creating something beautiful and useful, of advancing a cause or providing a service, is much greater than the pleasure of spending money in an attempt to compensate ourselves for an unfulfilling life. Having rewarding work also makes it much easier to love ourselves; indeed, it is the essence of self-loving.

In our culture, we experience lack and emptiness caused by the loneliness of separation from other people, nature, ourselves, and spirit. Trained from an early age to be consumers, we try to fill that lack with material possessions. If we could live in greater harmony with nature, we might recognize that our needs are really quite simple. Once we let go of status symbols and expensive diversions and learn to find enjoyment in creativity rather than consumption, we might feel much more fulfilled. According to Matthew Fox, our throats are the energy center through which our creativity is normally expressed. By stuffing ourselves with food and other consumer goods, we choke off our natural creative expression. Even while knowing all this, I catch myself thinking, "If I just had a computer with more memory, my life would be so much easier." Part of me still falls for the idea that my salvation will come from technology.

We live in a land of material abundance. Yet, as Mother Teresa once observed, the greatest disease in the United States is loneliness. Our very real experience of scarcity of love and approval leads to a generalized belief in scarcity. We engage in all sorts of addictive behavior to try to fill the void: consuming too much food, alcohol, drugs; mindlessly watching TV; compulsive sex, shopping, or overworking.

The act of giving, in contrast to getting and consuming, sends a message to our inner selves that we are experiencing abundance: "I must already have this, or I wouldn't be giving it away."

Embracing what we do want enables us to let go of what we don't really want. Gandhi wrote:

> As long as you derive inner help and comfort from anything, you should keep it. If you were to give it up in a mood of self-sacrifice or out of a stern sense of duty, you would continue to want it back, and that unsatisfied want would make trouble for you. Only give up a thing when you want some other condition so much that the thing no longer has any attraction for you.

Giving away what no longer serves us also makes more room for what does. Giving things away is a form of purification. It cleanses our immediate environment of excess "stuff," and releases an attachment to the material world. When I give away items such as clothing or books, it doesn't necessarily mean I'm making room for other material things to come in, like creating space in the closet for new clothes. Instead, the act of giving or letting go works on a broader and deeper level, allowing new ideas, new people, and new energies to come into my life. If I do yearn for some different outfits than the ones I have, I can buy second-hand clothes with a cleaner conscience than new ones, knowing that valuable resources did not have to be used and no one had to toil in a sweatshop to clothe me.

A vegetarian diet is easier on the planet than a meat-based one. John Robbins, in his well-researched book, *Diet for a New America,* makes a powerful case for vegetarianism. To meet our protein needs, it is about sixteen times less efficient to grow grain and use it to fatten livestock than to eat the grain ourselves. Chickens raised in factory farms have their beaks cut off to prevent them from pecking each other to death in their overcrowded cages, and rainforests are destroyed to graze cattle. According to the Sierra Club, American livestock generate 2.7 trillion pounds of manure per year, which has polluted 35,000 miles of rivers in twenty-two states and contaminated groundwater in over seventeen states; it isn't just a few hog farms in a North Carolina flood-plain. John Robbins' book cites these data: The average American man's risk of death from a heart attack is 50 percent; by eliminating meat, he can reduce that risk to 15 percent. A woman who eats meat daily is nearly four times more likely to get breast cancer than a woman who eats little or no meat; other cancers show similar patterns. Vegetarianism is like the Heimlich maneuver: It pops the meat out of our mouths before we die from it.

Despite years of espousing simpler living and attempting to place human connection above material goals, I received a painful demonstration of how much I was still stuck in my old patterns. In helping my 82-year-old mother prepare to move to a smaller place, I was giving more importance to getting her possessions efficiently sold, given away, or packed than to being caring and considerate of her timing and her needs. I grumbled and complained about how slow she was in deciding which of her books to give away. She said, with a mournful expression, "I'm saying goodbye to each of them." Most exasperating for me were the huge piles of solicitation letters, vitamin catalogs, magazines, and junk mail which she wanted to sort through. One evening I caught her going out to the recycle bin to see if she could retrieve something I'd tossed out. This whole process was very stressful for her, and as a result our relationship was strained. To my great sorrow, she passed away just a month after the move.

The Dalai Lama once said, "My religion is kindness." May I learn to choose kindness before efficiency.

In retrospect, I realize that one of the gifts I received from that trying time was a total-body conviction that accumulating stuff, even books and information, was not a path to happiness.

Joanna Macy, author of *Coming Back to Life*, has written of an approaching time she calls the "Great Turning": a time when humanity, through a shift in consciousness, turns away from the current path of self-destruction and embraces life-sustaining practices. I wonder whether there will be a "Great Purification," such as the Hopi prophecy predicts, in which all the toxicity we have generated will be transformed and cleansed, along with the mental patterns and thoughts that gave rise to it. Global warming, caused by our energy use, has already resulted in a vast increase in violent weather patterns, which may lead to severe global crop failures in coming years.

How might we stop short of the abyss? What is your favorite version of the story about how we humans stop destroying, and begin healing, our beautiful planet? I prefer to hold the image of each one of us restoring the environments where we live and work, as well as purifying our own bodies through cleaning up our diets and our thoughts.

For changing directions quickly, a bicycle is far better than a car.

There is growing poverty amid plenty in this unbalanced America, a scarcity of the physical essentials of life for many of our fellow citizens. We need to work for social and economic justice. But is it possible to abolish material poverty while we still have a scarcity of inner peace caused by our judgments of self and others? To heal that emptiness we need to strengthen and heal our relationships with each other and with all living things on the planet. The healing of all these relationships could be our most important work. When we are filled with spirit, our needs for ever more material "stuff" will be less than we ever believed.

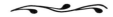

Ask yourself:
- What gives my life quality and makes it worth living?
- What would I need to change in my life, if gasoline suddenly became four times as expensive?
- What few possessions would I take if fleeing a fire, flood, or hurricane?

Connections

We are not healed alone.

—*A Course in Miracles*

If our primary path of continuing evolution has become the evolution of consciousness, then connections are crucial. Just as more abundant dendritic connections in the brain generate more intelligence, increased and deeper connections with people and other life forms enhance the development of consciousness. How ironic if, just as we realize the importance of these other creatures, they rapidly become extinct!

Joining

One of my favorite movies, *Groundhog Day,* shows the egotistical hero trying, with a great lack of success at first, to connect with a beautiful woman. At first he tries gimmicks like ordering her favorite drink as if it were his favorite too, or feigning an interest in French poetry. After much trial and error, and many opportunities to start over, he learns to meet each person with true empathy. Then, at last, he wins the fair lady (or perhaps she wins him).

To join with another is to enter their space, see things through their eyes. Doing this in a literal way can be useful. Try sitting next to the other person so that you view the world from the same perspective. The light and shade fall on you the same as on the other. Work as a team on problem solving (instead of from opposing sides). Put the problem in front of you where you can both look at it, not in between you. Work together on any project you can, starting with something of minor importance, where you currently are in agreement.

Make eye contact when possible. Match the other person's breathing pattern. Subtly match his or her body language. Behaving and moving in a way that mirrors another person (or animal or other being) brings us closer to their experience.

When our intention is to join, to resonate with another, we find ways to communicate; we enter into their world. Sometimes the only way we know to join is to do as they do, as with an autistic child—if he spins around, we spin too, to join with him in his world. It is not mimicry, but an act of respect. It's saying, "Your way is my way too, I'd like to share this experience with you." This approach dissolves the barriers between people. Barry Kaufman's book *Son-Rise* is the account of how he and his wife reached their autistic son and led him to recovery by starting with this sort of joining.

When I try to force someone to act the way I want, I can't see who she or he really is. I'm acting from my own need to validate my worthiness through making the other person do things my way.

My favorite story about joining is the tale of St. Francis and the wolf of Gubbio, as told by Murray Boto in his book *Francis: the Journey and the Dream*. Attending a retreat at a Franciscan center, I first heard the wolf story as it is usually told and then chanced to come across the version in Boto's book. According to the conventional story, the townspeople of Gubbio, who were terrorized by a ravenous wolf who attacked and ate children, asked St. Francis if he could intercede with the animal. The saint went to the wolf and made the sign of the cross. He spoke sternly to the wolf, asking it to desist from its attacks in the name of Christ. "Although you deserve to be punished for all the evil you have done, you will be given a chance to mend your ways. In return for ceasing your attacks, you will be fed by the townspeople."

In Boto's version of the story, however, Francis was quite fearful as he approached the wolf's lair. As he went, he thought about the parts of himself that were like the wolf: how he sometimes felt alone, misunderstood, hungry, aggressive. When he met the wolf, he first praised him for his strength. Then he acknowledged the wolf's ability to be a fierce protector for the townsfolk, and respectfully asked the wolf if he would be willing to serve in this way, in exchange for food, and to pledge nonviolence to the people of Gubbio. The wolf agreed, giving Francis his paw. Just as Francis begged for his food, so did the wolf go door to door and was fed. The wolf was transformed by his contact with the saint, and became well-loved by the townsfolk. It is said that an unusually large wolf's skull was found buried in the same church where Francis' remains were interred.

The story provides a wonderful model for how we can join with that which we fear or dislike the most, through honoring the strengths in that "other" and dissolving our false notions of separation and difference. Perhaps St. Francis was able to love and respect the wolf because he saw and accepted his own fierce, angry, ravenous aspects and did not have to put these parts of himself out of his heart. Honor and respect can work equally with other beings (whether wolves or people) and with parts of ourselves we have walled off and fear or distrust.

Poison oak was something I came to fear after a summer when I was almost continuously afflicted with itching, oozing rashes. It seemed that my relationship with this plant needed some attention. I spent some time honoring and then meditating next to a healthy specimen growing in a park. It occurred to me that I, too, am sometimes an irritant to people. I also realized that poison oak was doing a great job of keeping certain wild places protected from humans' encroachment. This is a value I can believe in. Since that time, I have suffered only very mild outbreaks. Interestingly, indigenous peoples are said to have been immune to the plant and used it as a medicinal to treat warts, ringworm, and even snake bite.

HERE ARE SOME QUESTIONS FOR REFLECTION:
- How is that "other" really like me?
- What positive qualities can I acknowledge in that "other"?
- How can I enlist his or her strengths?
- Can I accept the less lovable aspects of myself?

Community

> *Here, I brought you some heart soup. It's pretend soup,*
> *but it will give you real love. Because everyone needs*
> *love, and I just wanted to make sure you were getting*
> *enough.*   —David Wheeler, age 5

We are never really alone. We are part of the web of life, with all of nature as our relatives. Redwood trees have rather shallow roots, considering their great height. However, they never grow singly; they tend to form circles. What gives them stability is their roots interlocking with one another underground.

Consider the power of snowflakes. A snowflake or two may be quite insignificant; but when joined by thousands of others they can blanket a city, transforming it from dark ugliness to magical brightness and light.

Right now we need community more than ever before; we need to reach out past our seeming isolation, often engendered by our extreme busyness, and join hands with others. Community gives us safety and security, and holds us so that we can relax, open our hearts, and do our best work. A community is a place where people feel welcome in each other's homes. Ask yourself: "Where is my community?" We need to expand our circle of connection in ever-widening ripples, including animals and plants. You could hug a tree, talk to a houseplant, or stroke a cat. They are all our relations! As the song reminds us, "We are family." When we recognize and live this, we'll all be a lot less lonely.

Singing together in a group is an amazing way to experience unity and harmony. Pete Seeger had the gift of getting large audiences to sing in three-part harmony, which always brings an intense feeling of connection and closeness. Many spiritual teachers lead groups in singing; breathing together and making harmonious sounds is a powerful unifier. The Civil Rights movement had its songs; peace movements have theirs. People everywhere used to sing as they worked together. In Africa, they still do.

The greatest present we can give another is our *presence*: fully seeing and hearing and responding to that other person, creature, or plant in each moment.

If, like me, you don't have any children of your own, you can spend time with a friend's. Most children could use another caring adult in their lives, and your friend will be delighted. Many indigenous cultures turned over a good part of the education of children to the grandparents. These elders were not only the carriers of wisdom and tradition, but they also had more time since they were less involved in making a living. In our transient, mobile society, it is relatively rare for our society's grandparents to spend much time with their grandchildren, or for children to have aunts and uncles play a significant role in their care. I believe that a great role for the elders of our times would be teaching children to revere, restore, and protect the Earth.

Having a part-time child in my life has provided me with poetry, snuggling, and surprises. I've learned that fun and laughter are essential for well-being, and that destroying sand castles or towers of blocks can be as much fun as making them. I've learned that I can create whatever structure I like, limited only by my imagination. When we drew flowers together, David reminded me to draw the roots and the ground it grows on, not just the plant itself. It is a wonderful gift to see the world through his fresh, unconditioned viewpoint. I have experienced joy, love, and protectiveness arising within my heart.

One day David asked me to read him a story, which was about an old woman who resists adopting a puppy for fear she will outlive it. Afterwards, he quizzed me: "Did you get the moral of the story? Enjoy what you have, while you have it." David's offering of "heart soup" will always be precious in my memory. Every child I've ever met loves to be told stories starring him or her as the hero. They thrive on appreciation and acknowledgement of their wonderful qualities. Games, especially the same one with variations over time, are special; treasure hunts are one of the most delightful. A very favorite game is the baby animal game, which lets them pretend safely to be younger than they are and receive adult nurturing. I've fed many a baby bird.

As goes the heart, so goes the rhythm of the whole body. At the Institute for HeartMath in Boulder Creek, California, experiments have shown that the heart rate variability power-fully entrains the immune system. Even a few minutes of anger and frustration create an erratic heart pattern which can depress immune function for several hours. But when people feel appreciation and love, their heart rhythms become more coherent, and there is a marked increase in immune functioning.

We've forgotten that we are connected. So we've stopped talking to our neighbors, we've lost touch with old friends, we compete with other drivers instead of waving them ahead of us. Why not pay for the person behind you at the next bridge toll gate? Start a revolution. My friend Walt laughs with delight as he walks down a street popping quarters into expired parking meters. Give some food to a homeless person. Smile at a kid at the grocery store checkout. Silently bless a stranger on the street: "May you be well and happy." These small life-affirming actions are all ways to remind yourself that we are connected. We're like the islands in the Bay of Fundy: When the tide goes out, it's obvious we are all joined.

There is an inspiring story about a long line of people all waiting for guidance from a great master. Someone in the line, just as eager for wisdom from the master, discovered that the waiting was much easier to endure when giving service to the others in the line. Upon reaching the master he was told that, through his compassionate sharing, he had already received the wisdom he sought.

It's best for me to discover how and to whom I feel most comfortable giving, and start there, so that there is no experience of strain. Once the giving is in motion, the next little act of giving seems to flow more easily. Act as if you have plenty of whatever you are giving—whether it is love, a compliment, a smile, a wish for another's well-being, or material goods—and watch how your perspective changes.

Beware of giving from obligation. When we give from a closed heart, the other person receives only our resentment. I used to think I should get extra points for giving when I didn't really want to, and couldn't understand why people weren't a little more grateful. Giving from an open heart feels completely different both to the giver and to the recipient.

The more we give, the more we receive. We are setting into motion a great circle, as connected as breathing in and breathing out; we are joining in the grand natural cycle of life. To receive without giving, or to give without being able to receive in turn, would be like inhaling but never exhaling. When I was a health-care worker, I was often aware of how much my patients were taking care of me. As a respiratory therapist, I was quite fond of an elderly asthmatic lady who would arrive in the Emergency Room and, beaming at me as she gasped for air, inquire, "Are you married yet?"

In the Native American tradition of "potlatch," a huge giveaway was a powerful affirmation of abundance, of the giver and of nature itself.

Why not begin the new millennium with a great act of collective giving, such as cancelling all international debt? It could be humankind's final opportunity to transform from never-ending conflict to peace on earth.

> *Who understands what giving means must laugh at the idea of sacrifice.*   —A *Course in Miracles*

Epilogue

The sonnet with which I end this book was written when I was sixteen years old. It is about the risks and rewards of showing our true selves. Thank you for being willing to see me. Many blessings to you, and may your circle of healing and connection grow ever wider.

A BIRTH

When I stand up and speak, or in some act
Reveal myself, the living part of me,
Why does that self not bleed, or die in fact
Since it is thus revealed for all to see?
But those who witness are composed of dead
Expressions, make-up, gestures, and grimaces
Beneath which is the life, the life that fled
For fear, and hid itself from human faces.
So seeing me, when I had willingly
Laid bare my self, they felt within them rise
Their buried life, and answered gratefully
With joy of living contact in their eyes.
And is not love itself born of this sight:
One soul revealed, two in new life unite?

—C. H.

Resources

Recommended Readings

Ababio-Clottey, Aeeshah and Kokomon Clottey.
    Beyond Fear: Twelve Spiritual Keys to Racial Healing
Abram, David. *The Spell of the Sensuous*
Andrews, Ted. *Animal-Speak*
Arrien, Angeles. *The Four-fold Way*
Baldwin, Christina. *Calling the Circle*
Barasch, Mark. *The Healing Path: A Soul Approach*
    to Illness
Boone, J. Allen. *Kinship with All Life*
Boto, Murray. *Francis: The Journey and the Dream*
Brown, Molly Young. *Growing Whole*
Cahill, Sedonia. *The Ceremonial Circle*
Cameron, Julia. *The Artist's Way*
Capacchione, Lucia. *Recovery of Your Inner Child*
Carey, Ken. *Return of the Bird Tribes* and
    Flat Rock Journal
Carnes, Robin Dean and Sally Craig. *Sacred Circles: A*
    Guide to Creating Your Own Women's Spirituality
    Group
Casey, Caroline. *Making the Gods Work for You*
Cohen, Michael. *Connecting with Nature*
Cornell, Joseph. *Sharing Nature with Children*
Dossey, Larry. *Healing Words: The Power of Prayer and the*
    Practice of Medicine
Foundation for Inner Peace. *A Course in Miracles*
Frankl, Victor. *Man's Search for Meaning*

Garfield, Charles; Cindy Spring; & Sedonia Cahill.
      Wisdom Circles
Griffin, Donald. *Animal Minds*
Grossman, Warren. *To Be Healed by the Earth*
Hanh, Thich Nhat. *Miracle of Mindfulness* and
      Peace Is Every Step
Harner, Michael. *The Way of the Shaman*
Hill, Julia Butterfly. *The Legacy of Luna*
Huddleston, Peggy. *Prepare for Surgery, Heal Faster*
Kabat-Zinn, Jon. *Full Catastrophe Living*
Kaufman, Barry. *Son-Rise*
King, Serge Kahili. *Urban Shaman*
Lauck, Joanne. *The Voice of the Infinite in the Small*
Levine, Stephen. *Who Dies?* and *A Year to Live*
LeShan, Lawrence. *Cancer as a Turning Point*
Macy, Joanna and Molly Brown. *Coming Back to Life*
Mander, Jerry. *In the Absence of the Sacred*
McElroy, Susan. *Animals as Teachers and Healers*
Medicine Eagle, Brooke. *Buffalo Woman Comes Singing*
Metrick, Sydney and Renee Beck. *The Art of Ritual*
Myss, Caroline. *Anatomy of the Spirit*
Northrup, Christiane, M.D. *Women's Bodies,*
      Women's Wisdom
Pearsall, Paul, M.D. *The Heart's Code*
Peper, Erik and Cathy Holt. *Creating Wholeness:*
      A Self-Healing Workbook Using Dynamic
      Relaxation, Images and Thoughts
Quinn, Daniel. *Ishmael*
Rechtschaffen, Stephan. *Timeshifting*
Redfield, James. *The Celestine Vision*
Remen, Rachel Naomi. *Kitchen Table Wisdom*

Rinpoche, Sogyal. *The Tibetan Book of Living and Dying*
Robbins, John. *Reclaiming Our Health* and
    Diet for a New America
Rosenberg, Marshall. *Nonviolent Communication:*
    A Language of Compassion
Rossman, Martin. *Healing Yourself*
Sams, Jamie. *Medicine Cards* and *Sacred Path Cards*
Schneider, Meier. *My Life and Vision*
Seed, John et al. *Thinking Like a Mountain*
Sher, Barbara. *Wish-Craft* and *Live the Life You Love*
Shaffer, Carolyn and Kristin Anundsen. *Creating*
    Community Anywhere
Somé, Malidoma. *Ritual*
Starhawk, *The Spiral Dance*
Steindl-Rast, David. *Gratefulness, the Heart of Prayer*
Smith, Penelope. *Animals: Our Return to Wholeness* and
    Animal Talk
Stone, Hal and Sidra Winkelman. *Embracing Our Selves*
Swan, James. *Nature as Teacher and Healer*
Tolle, Eckhart. *The Power of Now*
Walsch, Neale Donald. *Conversations with God*
Weisberg, Alan. *Gaviotas: A Village to Reinvent the World*
Weil, Andrew. *Spontaneous Healing*
Wright, Machaelle Small. *Behaving as if the God in All*
    Life Mattered
Zimmerman, Jack and Virginia Coyle. *The Way of*
    Council

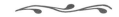

Videotherapy

Videotherapy is the practice of watching a certain videotape or movie to help you make a shift in a positive direction. Here is a list of some of my favorites, along with the problems they can address.

- *Brother Sun, Sister Moon* (the early life of St. Francis of Assisi): Feeling disconnected from nature, from other people, or from spirit
- *The Mission* or *Spitfire Grill:* Oppressed by guilt over the past
- *Koyanisqatsi* or *Walkabout:* Needing perspective on cultural imbalance
- *Groundhog Day:* Stuck in negative habits, not living in the present
- *Harold and Maude* or *King of Hearts:* Difficulty finding joy in life, or finding your own uniqueness
- *Housekeeping:* Perfectionism
- *Mr. Holland's Opus:* Stuck in the wrong job, not feeling creative
- *The Year of Living Dangerously:* If you think you were dealt an unfair hand, or see yourself as lacking
- *Microcosmos:* Lack of appreciation for insects and nematodes
- *The Secret Garden:* Self pity and illness; nature as healer
- *Ikiru* (To Live): Lack of purpose in life
- *It's a Wonderful Life:* Suicidal feelings, low self-worth
- *Lost Horizon:* Seeking right livelihood; utopia
- *Red Beard:* How emotions and life stories affect health
- *The Horse Whisperer:* Needing to learn trust and heal from trauma

- *Patch Adams* and *The Doctor:* Disillusion with the medical profession
- *Grand Canyon:* Feeling disconnected from other people and oneself; racial conflict; need for guidance
- *The Fisher King; King of Hearts;* also *Fearless:* Need for new perspectives on what is crazy
- *Life is Beautiful:* Needing humor in a very grim situation
- *The Straight Story:* Lack of cohesive family ties
- *Parenthood:* For overly achievement-oriented parents
- *The Secret of Roan Innish:* Understanding interspecies links
- *Man Facing Southeast* and *Jesus of Montreal:* Looking for the Christ amongst us

Audiotapes

- Holt, Cathy, *Kindness to the Body* (See order form at the back of the book)
- Peper and Holt. *Tapes to Accompany Creating Wholeness* (set of five relaxation and imagery tapes)
- Huddleston, Peggy. *Prepare for Surgery, Heal Faster*

I recommend any tapes by:
- Belleruth Naparstek (healing, surgery)
- Emmett Miller (relaxation, healing specific conditions)
- Martin Rossman, M.D. (guided imagery)
- Jon Kabat-Zinn (body scan relaxation; basic yoga)
- Angeles Arrien (healing stories)
- Brooke Medicine Eagle (*Healing through Ritual Action; Moontime; The Beauty Way;* and more)

Additional Resources

The *Self-Help Sourcebook* is the most complete resource outside of the Internet for finding and forming self-help groups. It is a publication of:
The American Self-Help ClearingHouse
St. Clare's–Riverside Medical Center
25 Pocono Road
Denville, N.J. 07834
(201) 625-9053

The NorthWest Earth Institute offers discussion courses for small groups: *Voluntary Simplicity, Deep Ecology, Choices for Sustainable Living*, and *Discovering a Sense of Place*. Affiliates exist in many states outside the northwest. For information on how to initiate a course in your workplace, faith community, or neighborhood, contact:
NorthWest Earth Institute
506 SW 6th Avenue, Suite 1100
Portland, OR 97204
(503) 227-2807
www.nwei.org

ABOUT THE AUTHOR

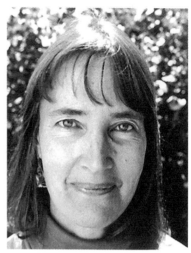

CATHY HOLT
is a holistic health educator and environmental activist. She co-authored a previous book and tape series called *Creating Wholeness: A Self-Healing Workbook Using Dynamic Relaxation, Images, and Thoughts*, with Erik Peper, Ph.D., and is a contributor to *EarthLight* magazine. A graduate of Radcliffe College, she received her Master's in Public Health from the University of California, Berkeley. As a biofeedback therapist, she has taught self-regulation skills to many clients with stress-related disorders and occupational injuries. She has also taught in hospitals, junior colleges, adult education centers, and JFK University's Graduate School of Holistic Health Studies. Her activism in the movements for peace, renewable energy, occupational health, deep ecology, and voluntary simplicity spans three decades. She currently assists patients in preparing for surgery and leads workshops on letting nature heal.

If you liked this book and wish to pass it on to a friend, check with your local bookstore or online bookseller, or use the order form on reverse.

An audiocassette tape, *Kindness to the Body,* was made to accompany the book. It contains guided relaxation and imagery to help you nurture your body and contact your inner wisdom. See options for ordering on reverse.

Excerpts from the book, ordering information, and newsbits can be found at
www.TalkingBirdsPress.com

Order Form

Options for ordering a copy of this book and/or the companion audiotape by Cathy Holt:

- Fax this form to (510) 835-2765
- Call 1-800-404-9492 (credit card only)
- Send check and order form to
  Talking Birds Press, P. O. Box 13073, Berkeley, CA 94712

Please send me:

The Circle of Healing
_____ copies at $14.95 each   _____

Kindness to the Body audiotape
_____ copies at $9.95 each   _____

Book and tape combination
_____ sets at $24 each   (Save)   _____

Sales tax
(Add 8.25 percent for products shipped to California addresses:
$1.23 for one book, .82 for one tape, 1.98 for one set.)   _____

Shipping/Handling (priority 2-day mail, U.S.)   _____
$4 for the first book, add $2 per additional book
$5 for one book/audiotape set, add $2 per additional set
$3.50 for one audiotape, add $1 per additional tape

Total: _____

Ship to:

_____
Name

_____
Address

_____   _____   _____
City   State   Zip

Payment: ☐ Check to Talking Birds Press
            ☐ MasterCard ☐ VISA

_____   _____
Card Number   Expiration Date

_____
Name on Card

_____
Signature